# Natural Healing

## with

# Cell Salts

# NATURAL HEALING

## WITH

# CELL SALTS

Skye Weintraub, N.D.

The information in this book is for educational purposes only and is not recommended as a means of diagnosing or treating an illness. All matters concerning physical and mental health should be supervised by a health practitioner knowledgeable in treating that particular condition. Neither the publisher nor author directly or indirectly dispense medical advice, nor do they prescribe any remedies or assume any responsibility for those who choose to treat themselves.

Woodland Publishing, Inc.
P.O. Box 160
Pleasant Grove, UT 84062
(800) 777-2665

Cover design by Kevn Lambson

ISBN 1-885670-29-X

If unavailable at your local bookstore, this book may be ordered from the publisher at the above phone number and address.

"ye are the salt of the earth . . ."

# Contents

# FOREWORD

Every physician has close at hand several well-worn reference books that are essential to their practice. In my office one of those books is the first edition of Natural Healing with Cell Salts, compiled by Dr. Skye Weintraub, N.D.

Dr. Weintraub introduced me to cell salt therapy when we worked together as student clinicians at National College of Naturopathic Medicine. The cell salts have been a fundamental part of my practice. They are simple, specific, and effect a cure by restoration of function on a cellular level. The results are long lasting. I have seen profound results in a wide variety of physical and emotional conditions.

I use cell salts with a majority of my clients and find them particularly useful with children. I encourage the parents of my young clients to keep all the cell salts on hand at home as a first aid kit. This will enable them to have remedies available when their child wakes up sick in the middle of the night. Animals also respond well to cell salts. Administer the tablets by dissolving them in water and applying with an eye dropper.

Dr. Weintraub's repertoire is useful for both trained health care practitioners and lay people. I am grateful to her for having created this resource, and my hope is that it will promote broader use of these simple and remarkable remedies.

Louise N. Edwards, N.D., L.Ac.

# INTRODUCTION TO CELL SALT THERAPY

A key researcher investigating the many roles of minerals in the human body was Dr. W. H. Schuessler, M.D., of Oldenburg, Germany. It was fascinating to him that natural substances could cure disease. He studied the work of another great 19th-century thinker, Virchow, who in 1858, announced that the body is a collection of cells and medical treatment should be directed toward healing the individual cell.

The "cell theory" of Virchow made perfect sense to Dr. Schuessler. By 1873, he was analyzing blood from humans as well as the ashes after death. After isolating minerals from these various tissues, he knew that minerals were an integral part of the body. Twelve mineral compounds were discovered and he called them "cell salts," or "tissue salts."

As Dr. Schuessler researched the minerals further, he felt that if the body became deficient in any of these important minerals an abnormal or diseased condition occurred. He studied the various symptoms and discovered which minerals were lacking in his patients. When the correct minerals were supplied the abnormal or diseased symptom(s) decreased or disappeared, if they were curable at all. It was also important to give the correct amount and frequency. With the proper cell salts added to the sick cells of the body, the abnormality corrected and the body healed itself. This was the beginning of Dr. Schuessler's biochemic system of medicine.

This biochemic theory has withstood the test of time. Even with far more sophisticated laboratory equipment available, the simplicity of cell salts is just as valid today as it was one hundred years ago when Dr. Schuessler developed them. Actually, they have improved. There is a better understanding of how they work and manufacturers make high-quality cell salts for general use.

Cell salts are more popular than ever. They can be prescribed safely and are an inexpensive way for people to self-treat many of the ills that exist. You can experiment to find out which one you need without fear of damaging your health. This 19th-century discovery is still useful for health concerns today.

Dr. Schuessler also believed that the twelve cell salts contained all the active ingredients used by traditional homeopathy. Using cell salts simplifies the practice of homeopathic medicine. Whether we know it or not we find the components of cell salts widely throughout nature: from the food we eat, the earth we walk on, the rocks, the soil, and vegetation. Their concentrations are high in the mineral springs we visit for health-restoring properties.

The cells of our body contain minute but perfectly balanced quantities of water, as well as organic and inorganic substances. Well-nourished cells provide us with the building blocks of health. When we properly assimilate nutrients, these cells replenish each day. Specific cells build up specific areas of the body. The inorganic salts that make up these cells help to determine the differences in tissues and organs. The correct balance of these tissue cell salts must be maintained for proper structure and function of each tissue and organ.

The body provides an accurate indication of balance by functioning in perfect harmony and being healthy and symptom-free. If the cells do not receive their proper nourishment or when they cannot rid themselves of toxic waste, a disease process will begin. In due time, the automatic alarm system activates symptoms.

The success of biochemical cell salt therapy lies in accurately linking a person's symptoms with the appropriate tissue cell salt. Symptoms occur in a variety of forms and are a guide to the nature of the body's deficiency and to the correct treatment required. How and where they occur will help you decide the correct tissue cell salt. Often, you need more than one. The proper dose replenishes the cell salt supply and restores tissue or organ function.

# HOW TO SELECT AND USE CELL SALTS

When you carefully note the most prominent symptoms, one or more remedies will usually closely match these symptoms. If you have a sore throat, you would turn to the throat section. Under the heading, "sore," find the best individual symptom(s), and give all remedies listed. Some ailments, especially acute ones, may change during a treatment. In such cases, change the remedies as your symptoms change, at each successive stage of recovery. Your lack of symptoms verifies a restored healthy body balance.

The cell salt remedies described in this book are meticulously extracted from living plants in an alcohol process. Manufacturers pulverized the natural mineral substances and blend them with milk sugar to make them more palatable. Many potencies are available, but the 3X and 6X are the best for home use. The most generally useful potency is 6X. See "Directions for Use" for a more detailed description on the use of cell salts.

Cell salts provide inorganic elements in a form that ensures their transportation and assimilation into the body. Usually it is not advisable to allow the salts to pass directly through the digestive tract, because digestion sometimes fails to liberate the inorganic substances from the organic parts. Cell salts absorb directly into the blood stream through the osmotic process. Place the tablets under the tongue to dissolve because this is where the capillary beds lie close to the surface of the skin.

Biochemical cell salt therapy also works with great success in the treatment of domestic animals. Their symptoms are a guide to the correct remedy needed. Animals usually respond quickly, but if symptoms persist, consult a veterinarian.

# MATERIA MEDICA OF THE CELL SALT REMEDIES

## 1. Calc Fluor

SYNONYMS....Calcium Fluoride, Calcaria Flurica

COMMON NAME....Fluoride of lime, Fluorspar

This remedy occurs in nature as the mineral fluorspar. The combining of calcium and fluoride produces a remedy with healing powers shown by neither of the constituents alone. A disturbance in the equilibrium of the molecules of the cell creates a relaxed condition. This causes an interference with absorption and can lead to hardening and swelling of the tissues. Such a disturbance causes the enlargement of blood vessels that appear as hemorrhoidal tumors, varicosities, enlarged veins, vascular tumors, and swollen and hardened glands.

Calc Fluor is useful in treating many ailments of the bones and teeth. It is part of the surface of bones and tooth enamel. It is in the walls of blood vessels, and in muscular and connective tissue.

Elastic fibers contain as a prime ingredient Calc Fluor. In the body, Calc Fluor is useful in treating diseases of the skin and blood vessels. The restorative property of this remedy is in its ability to maintain elasticity of the tissues. Use it for uterine displacements, teeth loose in their sockets, sluggish circulation, muscular weakness, and ailments of tendons, ligaments, and fibrous tissue. Associated with this elastic tissue builder are cracks in the skin, especially in the hands and toes.

## 2. Calc Phos

SYNONYMS....Calcium Phosphate, Calcarea Phosphoricum

COMMON NAME....Phosphate of Lime

Because it is a major constituent of bones, Calc Phos is also a chief builder of bone tissue, and the principal salt deficient in diseases of bone structure. All the cells and fluids of the body contain this cell salt. There is a need for Calc Phos to promote healthy cellular activity and to restore tone to weakened organs and tissues.

Give Calc Phos for its restorative powers after acute diseases and infections. It has the capacity to build up new blood cells and can therefore treat many forms of anemia. Essential to the proper growth and general all-around nutrition of the body, Calc Phos is the cell salt for being generally run-down. Use it for children who are not developing properly. Even when symptoms show a need for another cell salt, this remedy is often advisable, because it can intensify the action of other cell salts. Calc Phos is indicated in the elderly, where regenerative function decreases in the nervous tissue.

An insufficient supply results in defective nutrition, imperfect growth, and decay. It is of great importance after drains on the system and during malassimilation. Use it for infants' teething problems, inherited weaknesses, and disease tendencies. Calc Phos especially helps young, rapidly growing children. Use it again at puberty, as well as in old age.

Calc Phos and Mag Phos are the two remedies for cramps and spasms. Use both for most kinds of cramps. Take 5 tablets of each cell salt and dissolve in hot water. Sip the liquid frequently, holding it under the tongue for approximately one minute. Repeat every 3 hours.

## 3. Calc Sulph

SYNONYMS....Calcium Sulphate, Calcarea Sulphate

COMMON NAMES....Sulphate of Lime, Gypsum, Plaster of Paris

Found in nature as anhydrite, gypsum, alabaster and selenite, this remedy works well with Silica as a healer of wounds. It is a chief builder of epithelial tissue and furnishes the cohesive substance to sustain the integrity of the body's tissues. As a skin remedy, it is important in the formation of new skin and as an eliminator of waste materials. If there is a deficiency, suppuration will result, or a discharge of pus.

Considered a great blood purifier and healer, Calc Sulph helps the liver with the removal of waste products from the blood stream. Use in cases arising from impurities in the blood stream, such as minor skin ailments, acne, and pimples during adolescence. Calc Sulph's action works just the opposite of Silica. Silica hastens the process of suppuration, while this remedy closes up a process that has continued too long. It can clean out the tissue that is suppurating by causing it to discharge readily. This action is important to the healing process.

This tissue builder helps for the third stage of catarrh, bronchitis, lung disease, boils, ulcers, abscesses or exudations from any part of the body. It has a purifying and cleansing effect throughout the system making it important in the fight against new infections. Don't use Calc Sulph below the 6X potency.

# 4. Ferr Phos

SYNONYMS....Ferrum Phosphate, Iron Phosphate

COMMON NAME....Phosphate of Iron

This is the primary biochemical first-aid remedy because it carries oxygen throughout the body and strengthens the walls of the blood vessels, especially the arteries. It is the cell salt most concerned with the blood because it is part of hemoglobin, the substance that takes up oxygen from the inhaled air and carries it through the bloodstream to all parts of the body. Because of Ferr Phos's important role in carrying oxygen, it is recommended in nearly all conditions.

It can stop the flow of blood in abnormal hemorrhage. You can control mild hemorrhage by applying the powder topically to the wound. In conditions of fever and inflammation, there is usually a Ferr Phos deficiency. Give this remedy in the early stages of most acute disorders, and again at frequent intervals until the symptoms subside. It is excellent in ailments of the elderly and for children.

# 5. Kali Mur

SYNONYMS....Kali Muriaticum, Potassium Chloride

COMMON NAME....Chloride of Potash

Kali Mur occurs naturally in the mineral carnallite. It works very much like Kali Sulph, but its action is more subtle. Kali Mur is an essential constituent of muscles, nerve cells, blood, and brain cells. It is the mineral worker of the blood that forms protein fiber and fibrin. When the body contains the correct amount of Kali Mur, fibrin is functional, and deficiency symptoms do not manifest. A deficiency causes fibrin to be thrown off as a thick, white discharge.

In chronic ailments it is especially helpful in treating severe inflammation. Kali Mur can help destroy waste material when the body is fighting off a fever or infection. Because it is a building agent, give this remedy to aid the process of convalescing and rebuilding health. Kali Mur helps to develop new vitality and energy.

This inorganic salt is the remedy for sluggish conditions. When used for the liver, take it in the 12X dose three times a day. This is the same amount of Kali Mur that occurs naturally in a healthy blood cell. Involved with the production of saliva, it is important in the early stages of digestion. Use for the first-aid treatment of burns, as a blood conditioner, and for such ailments as coughs, colds, chills, and bronchitis. Kali Mur can retard the secretion mechanism of the body. The throat and Eustachian tube are the organs most influenced by Kali Mur.

# 6. Kali Phos

SYNONYMS....Kali Phosphoricum, Potassium Phosphate

COMMON NAME....Phosphate of Potash

Kali Phos is the remedy for jangled nerves. As a nerve nutrient, it has become essential in the treatment of nervous conditions. Used around the world as a natural tranquilizer, it has helped people who have suffered from such problems as grief, despair, and sorrow for long periods of time. Kali Phos appears to restore direction and order to both the mind and the body.

Being a necessary part of nervous tissue, it is important in the treatment of irritating skin ailments, such as shingles. It is part of animal fluids and tissues, especially the brain, nerves, muscles and blood cells. Kali Phos powerfully influences bodily functions and is indispensable to the formation of tissues, the oxidation process, and other chemical transformations in the blood.

While Ferr Phos helps to regulate the external breathing of cells, Kali Phos regulates the internal breathing in the exchange of gases. They both carry oxygen, and some biochemists believe that Kali Phos can carry oxygen to places where Ferr Phos cannot. This important cell salt is antiseptic and hinders the decay of tissues. Kali Phos is a brain builder and the basis of brain or nerve fluid. Indications for this remedy are a lack of nerve power, prostration, nervous headaches, loss of mental vigor, depression, student brain-fog, rapid decomposition of the blood, as a stress remedy for shock, etc. Kali Phos operates well with Mag Phos in the restoration of nerve fibers. This cell salt is one of the greatest healing agents known to humankind.

## 7. Kali Sulph

SYNONYMS....Kali Sulphuricum, Potassium Sulfate

COMMON NAMES....Sulphate of Potash

This inorganic cell salt occurs naturally in lava. It has a beneficial effect on the respiration of the body by working with Ferr Phos to help blood carry oxygen to all the cells. It also aids in conditions of the lungs, sinuses, and the bronchi. Known as the anti-friction cell salt, Kali Sulph acts like a lubricant of parts. Use this cell salt in the late stages of all inflammations.

Kali Sulph is very important for healthy skin and is the functional remedy for diseases of the epidermis and epithelium. It helps build new skin cells where the old ones die or become damaged due to disease. Prescribe Kali Sulph with other indicated remedies for skin problems.

Kali Sulph is a builder and distributor of oil made in the body. A deficiency of this remedy causes oil in the system to become non-functional. It becomes thick and clogs the pores, or presents as a sticky, yellowish discharge from the skin, mucous membranes, or any orifice of the body. This oil substance can discharge from any glandular swelling, abscess, cancer, etc.

## 8. Mag Phos

SYNONYMS....Magnesium Phosphate

COMMON NAMES....Phosphate of Magnesium

This antispasmodic cell salt is a remarkable remedy. As part of the white fibers of muscles and nerves, it supplements the action of Kali Phos concerning the nervous system, and as a brain salt. Its primary function is in correcting violent ailments, especially spasms. Being a nerve stabilizer, it reduces spasmodic darting pains such as those found in sciatica, or neuralgia. Mag Phos works well with Calc Phos for most kinds of cramps.

Deficiencies of Mag Phos result in conditions that manifest symptoms such as flatulence, convulsions, and other nervous disturbances. All the phosphate cell salts help with ailments of the nerves. The organs of affinity are especially the muscles and the heart. This important mineral insures rhythmic and coherent movement to the muscular tissue, and is a great remedy for nearly all heart problems.

Although found abundantly in cereal grains, most people don't get enough magnesium in their diet. The milling process of the grain removes the precious outer layers of magnesium-rich fibers. For speedy symptomatic relief of spasmodic ailments, dissolve 1-2 tablets under the tongue. Then dissolve 2-3 tablets in some hot water, taken in sips. Hold the liquid under the tongue for a minute each time. The 6X potency is usually sufficient.

## 9. Nat Mur

SYNONYMS....Natrum Muriaticum, Sodium Chloride

COMMON NAMES....Chloride of Soda, Common Table Salt

Occurring abundantly in nature, nearly everywhere, Nat Mur is the water distributor. It is present in every fluid and solid part of the body. This remedy is also present in intercellular fluid. In the proper ratio Nat Mur results in protective action of the cell membrane. The prime function of Nat Mur is to maintain a proper degree of moisture throughout the system. This remedy regulates the degree of moisture within the cells by attracting water to the body tissues. Nat Mur reaches the blood through the epithelial cells of the mucous membranes, and reaches the various cells where it provides the needed moisture.

Exceptional dryness or excessive moisture in any part of the body usually shows the need for Nat Mur. There may be a craving for salt, but table salt is not helpful. It can't be adequately absorbed by the body for these conditions. It needs to be prepared in homeopathic doses. The organs in the body most influenced by Nat Mur are the kidneys and sinuses. This remedy is an anti-histamine. Use it for relief of hay fever conditions. It also relieves imbalances of the lymphatic system, blood, spleen, and the mucous membrane lining of the alimentary canal.

## 10. Nat Phos

SYNONYMS....Natrum Phosphoricum, Sodium Phosphate

COMMON NAMES....Phosphate of Soda

This remedy is the great acid balancer. As a biochemical antacid, it regulates the acid-base balance in the stomach. Use Nat Phos when symptoms of acidity are present such as dyspepsia, digestive upsets, and heartburn. Another key function of Nat Phos is its ability to help in the assimilation of fats. Many antacids taken for stomach upset contain bicarbonate of soda. Because of the high sodium content, bicarbonate of soda can cause the formation of kidney stones, recurrent urinary tract infections, and problems in people with incipient heart trouble or kidney problems.

Nat Phos is the principal remedy for ailments arising from an acid condition in the blood, such as rheumatism. This remedy is indicated whenever conditions result from an excess of acid in the system. It neutralizes the acid. It also acts upon the bowels, glands, lungs, and abdominal organs to bring the system back into balance.

Many intense emotional symptoms manifest because of acid conditions of the blood, such as hate, envy, criticism, jealousy, competition, selfishness, suicide, and murder. Chemical poisons from too much acid in the body can cause irritation to the brain cells.

## 11. Nat Sulph

SYNONYMS....Natrum Sulphuricum, Sodium Sulphate

COMMON NAMES....Sulphate of Soda, Glauber's Salt

This inorganic salt occurs abundantly in nature. You find it in sea water and saline springs. In the body it is in the intercellular fluids, liver, and pancreas where Nat Sulph adjusts the density of the fluids. It can regulate the carrying of water away from the body tissues and help to eliminate many disease processes. Nat Sulph also acts to remove normal wastes from the cells. Use this cell salt when there are symptoms such as chills, malaria, influenza, watery infiltration, and other conditions where there is a need to regulate the excretion of superfluous water.

Nat Sulph is also important as a liver salt. It controls the healthy function of the liver, and is helpful for any liver problem, such as biliousness. Nat Sulph stimulates the epithelial cells of the bile ducts, pancreas, and intestinal canal. It returns normal secretions to these organs and stimulates their nerves. This cell salt is also useful in the later stages of digestion.

## 12. Silica

SYNONYM....Silica Oxide

COMMON NAMES....Pure Flint, Quartz, Silicious Earth

Silica is abundant throughout the vegetable kingdom, especially in grasses, palms, and grains. This remedy cleanses and eliminates waste. It helps the body to throw off non-functional organic matter and is called the "homeopathic surgeon." Silica is a profound tissue salt. It can create a passage to the surface for the discharge of pus, and to rid the body of this impurity. It can often initiate the healing process by promoting suppuration and breaking up pathological accumulation, such as in abscesses and boils. Since Silica restores activity to the skin, and aids in the cleansing process it helps to cure chronic skin conditions.

This tissue cleanser is a slow worker, but its action is deep and long lasting. It is helpful for impure blood conditions and chronic sepsis. Silica acts as an insulator for the nerves; influences the bones, joints, glands, skin, and mucous membranes; and is associated with ailments that create pus formation. It is a basic nutrient of the skin, hair, and nails. Silica works well for constitutions that are imperfectly nourished because of deficient assimilation. Sensitive patients who are always chilly may need Silica.

# 4

# DIRECTIONS FOR USE

Take biochemical cell salts with perfect safety. They do not produce unwanted side-effects, conflict with other medicines, and are non-addictive. Even babies and small children can take them with complete safety. Cell salts are usually available from health food stores in the form of tablets. Some health practitioners make them available in liquid form.

For the greatest effectiveness, place the tablets under the tongue, and allow them to dissolve. This lets the dose of cell salts bypass the stomach, which assures that the remedy or remedies will travel quickly and undamaged to the cells that are diseased or injured. Avoid gum or tobacco or strongly flavored substances near the time you take the cell salts. Do not drink liquids or eat foods for at least 15 minutes before or after taking the tablets. If you need quick relief, dissolve the tablets in a cup of hot water and sip often. Hold the liquid under the tongue for about a minute for maximum absorption. If a reaction occurs, such as an aggravation of symptoms, it is best to let the symptoms subside before repeating the dose.

If more than one remedy is strongly indicated, you can mix the different cell salts together. Never touch any of the cell salt tablets with your fingers. Use a clean spoon to remove them from the bottle and then place them under the tongue.

For external use dissolve 2-3 tablets of each indicated remedy in a tablespoon of hot water. After they have completely dissolved, dip a cotton swab in the liquid and dab it on the affected place. Apply the cell salts in powdered form to areas needed for first-aid conditions, such as cuts and wounds. Follow external applications with the internal treatment of cell salts.

Most homeopathic remedies can be stored for many years when you close the bottles tightly and kept in dry areas free from light, radiation, and away from strong odors. There are substances that can cause the cell salts to become non-functional. These substances are coffee, alcohol, aromatics such as mint in your toothpaste, and strongly spiced food. Avoid during treatment. This also includes Tiger balm, Ben-Gay, Vick's, Noxema, and other products containing camphor. Avoid tobacco and its smoke, especially containing menthol. Do not expose yourself to strong odors such as Lyosol, fresh paint, and eucalyptus used in steam baths.

Several other cautions are important during treatment: avoid handling the tablets because of contamination; never expose the medicines to direct sunlight; don't eat raw garlic during treatment; don't expose the cell salts to x-ray in airports; don't sleep under electric blankets; and avoid caffeine in coffee, colas, and chocolate.

Hold tablets under the tongue until they dissolve. For small children and pets, it may be easier to dose by dissolving the tablets in a little water first. Then squirt the liquid inside the lip or under the tongue. Liquid homeopathic remedies are available from some health-care practitioners and used in a similar manner as the tablet form. Continue the indicated salt(s) for several days after the symptoms clear.

# Dosage

**Adult**....................Take 3-4 tablets three to four times a day. Take 10-15 drops of a liquid remedy three times a day.

**Children**...............Take 2 tablets three to four times a day. Take 3 drops of a liquid remedy three times a days.

**Infant**..................1 tablet may be dissolved in warm water three times a day and sipped. Hold each sip under the tongue as long as possible. The liquid can be placed in the belly button three times a day; hold in area for about 5 minutes.

Chronic cases: Take tablets three to four times a day. The remedy or remedies may have to be taken for a month or longer.

Acute cases of sudden onset: Take one dose 1 to 2 hours apart and decrease frequency as symptoms improve.

Acute, severe, or painful cases: Dose every 15 minutes to an hour, and decrease frequency with improvement.

Less acute cases: Give the remedy hourly, and decrease the frequency as symptoms improve.

Give all the cell salt remedies listed following the indicated symptom(s).

# REPERTOIRE

## ABDOMEN

abscess....Silica
bloated....Mag Phos, Kali Sulph
burning, with sore pain in pit of stomach....Ferr Phos
cold feeling to the touch....Kali Sulph
colic....Mag Phos
cramps....Mag Phos
distended....Mag Phos
empty feeling about navel....Calc Phos
feels cold to the touch....Kali Sulph
flabby, large, even when person is generally thin....Calc Phos
flatulent distention of the abdomen....Nat Mur
full sensation, due to gas....Mag Phos, Nat Sulph
hardness....Nat Phos
hernia

    general, in....Calc Phos
    incarcerated, inflamed....Ferr Phos
    inflammation and fever....Ferr Phos

large....Silica
looseness, hereditary, in elderly women....Nat Sulph
pain

    colicky, flatulent....Kali Sulph
    cutting....Ferr Phos, Mag Phos, Nat Sulph
    navel, around, causing crying....Calc Phos, Mag Phos
    relieved by pressure, warmth, rubbing....Mag Phos

pendulous....Calc Phos
sinking sensation

    epigastrium, in, and about navel....Calc Phos
    problems with digestion, and....Calc Phos

stimulates intestinal, liver and pancreatic secretions....Nat Sulph
sunken....Calc Phos
swelling of....Kali Mur
swollen....Kali Phos, Kali Mur, Mag Phos
tender to touch....Kali Mur
tense and tympanic....Kali Sulph
waist, cannot bear tight clothing around....Nat Sulph
weakness in epigastrium....Kali Phos
worse symptoms with rich and fatty foods....Kali Mur

ABORTION (see Pregnancy and Labor)

ABSCESS

acidity, increased, with....Nat Phos
anus, about....Calc Sulph
beginning stage....Ferr Phos
chronic....Calc Phos, Silica
cleansing and healing, to help with....Calc Sulph
fistulous....Silica, Nat Sulph
gums (see also Gums)....Calc Fluor, Silica, Calc Sulph
heat and pain, with....Ferr Phos
inflammation, pain and throbbing....Ferr Phos
mature, helps abscess; when matter has formed....Calc Sulph
pharynx, of....Ferr Phos
psoas, of....Silica
ripen and suppurate, helps to....Silica
second stage, with swelling and discharge....Kali Mur
suppuration (see also Suppuration)
    clears up....Calc Sulph
    long standing....Calc Sulph
    promotes discharge of pus rendering the skin
        healthy....Silica
    shortens....Calc Sulph
swelling without pus formation; give in early stages....Ferr Phos,
    Kali Mur
tonsils (see also Tonsils)....Calc Sulph, Silica

ACCIDENTS (see also Injuries, First Aid)

muscles, strained; give every three hours (see also Strained)....Calc
    Fluor, Ferr Phos, Kali Mur
suppuration, long-standing (see also Suppuration)....Calc Sulph
wounds (see Wounds)

ACIDITY

acid conditions in general; take before meals; other indicated
    remedies should be given a few minutes later....Nat Phos
excessive; any symptoms of acidity....Nat Phos
neutralizer; ailments arising from an acid condition of the
    blood....Nat Phos
sensitive to....Mag Phos
stomach, acid; take before meals....Nat Phos

## ACNE

    Acne Rosacea....Kali Mur, Calc Phos, Silica, Nat Phos

    adolescent; precede with Silica....Calc Sulph

    chronic....Kali Mur, Calc Sulph, Calc Phos, Silica

    complexion, bad, earthy, with inclination to constipation; generally depressed in mind and body....Nat Mur

    eruptions on face, neck, shoulders; precede with Silica (see also Eruptions)....Calc Sulph

    puberty, especially during; menses too early and too free in young girls; much backache....Calc Phos

    pustules, watery (see also Pustules)....Nat Mur, Kali Mur, Ferr Phos

    swellings....Kali Mur

## ACUTE

    diseases, give after; it has restorative powers....Calc Phos

    disorders; give in the early stage and administered frequently until the inflammatory symptoms subside....Ferr Phos

## ADDICTION, morphine....Nat Phos

## ADDISON'S DISEASE....Nat Mur, Nat Sulph

## ADENOIDS....Calc Fluor, Calc Phos, Ferr Phos, Kali Mur

## ADHESIONS....Calc Fluor, Ferr Phos

## AGGRAVATES SYMPTOMS (see also Worse, Symptoms Become)

    atmosphere

        dusty....Kali Sulph

        salty....Nat Mur

    bites of insects....Nat Mur

    chilling of feet....Silica

    cold....Calc Phos, Mag Phos, Silica, Nat Phos, Nat Mur

    cold air....Kali Phos, Mag Phos

    dampness....Nat Sulph, Calc Fluor

    drafts....Calc Fluor, Mag Phos

    exercise, continued....Kali Phos

    exertion

        mental....Kali Phos, Nat Phos

        physical....Kali Phos, Nat Phos

    extremes of temperature; hot or cold....Calc Sulph

    foods

        bread....Nat Mur

fatty....Kali Mur
fish....Nat Sulph
fruit....Calc Phos
pastry....Kali Mur
rich....Kali Mur
watery foods....Nat Sulph
fresh air....Kali Sulph, Nat Phos
hot atmosphere, suffocative feeling in....Kali Sulph
lying
down....Kali Sulph
left side, on....Nat Sulph
moon, full and new; increases symptoms....Silica
motion....Calc Phos, Kali Mur, Ferr Phos
movement after rest....Kali Phos
noise....Kali Phos, Silica
open air, when in....Ferr Phos, Nat Phos, Silica
pressure....Silica
rest, after....Kali Phos
rising from sitting position....Kali Phos
sea bathing....Kali Mur
seashores....Nat Mur
standing still or lying down....Kali Sulph
thunderstorms, before and during....Silica, Nat Phos
touching....Mag Phos
warm room....Calc Sulph, Kali Sulph
water, washing or working in....Calc Sulph, Nat Sulph
weather
change of....Calc Phos, Calc Fluor
cold....Calc Fluor, Nat Mur, Kali Mur, Silica
damp....Nat Sulph, Calc Fluor, Calc Phos
dry becoming wet....Silica
wet....Nat Sulph
wet, becoming....Calc Sulph, Calc Phos

## AGING

ailments associated with....Ferr Phos
debilitated where there is inadequacy of spinster control and
dribbling....Calc Phos
elderly, excellent for ailments associated with....Ferr Phos, Calc
Phos
generally helpful to older people....Silica, Calc Fluor, Kali Mur

lubricating agent; helpful in older people who tend to lose lubrication in their skin....Kali Sulph

senility
> general, in....Kali Phos
> premature....Calc Phos, Kali Phos, Silica

AGITATED....Silica

AGUE....Nat Sulph (3X), Ferr Phos, Nat Mur, Kali Phos

ALCOHOLISM....Mag Phos

ALOPECIA (see also Hair)
areata....Kali Phos
bald spots; hair falling out....Calc Phos, Kali Sulph
dry hair and falls out; beard hair falls out....Nat Mur
fever, after....Calc Phos
healthy hair, for retaining....Silica
loss and thinning not connected to a fever....Calc Fluor, Silica
relieves baldness; there are some indications that this remedy may help in time take along with the patient's particular constitutional cell salt....Kali Sulph
senilis....Silica
whiskers, of....Nat Mur

AMELIORATES SYMPTOMS
applications
> cold....Ferr Phos
> heat....Mag Phos, Silica

bending double....Mag Phos
cold....Ferr Phos, Calc Fluor
company....Kali Phos
cool air, fresh....Kali Sulph
eating....Kali Phos, Nat Phos
evening....Nat Mur
excitement, cheerful....Kali Phos
fomentations....Calc Fluor
fresh air....Calc Sulph, Kali Sulph
friction....Mag Phos
getting up and slowly walking around, after....Kali Phos
heat....Silica, Mag Phos, Calc Fluor
lying down
> general, in....Silica, Calc Phos
> something hard, on....Nat Mur

mind, diversion of....Kali Phos
moist warmth....Silica
motion, gentle....Kali Phos
pressure....Mag Phos
rest....Calc Phos, Kali Phos
rubbings....Calc Fluor
salt....Nat Mur
walking
    general, in....Calc Sulph
    open air, in....Kali Sulph
warm, dry atmosphere....Calc Sulph, Nat Sulph
warm room....Silica
warmth....Calc Phos, Silica, Mag Phos
weather
    change of....Nat Sulph
    warm, dry....Nat Sulph, Calc Sulph
wrapping up head....Silica

## AMENORRHEA

anemia, along with mental depression and inclined to be constipated; after one month also give Calc Phos....Nat Mur
bilious symptoms, with....Nat Sulph
change of climate, with....Silica, Calc Phos
chill, due to....Ferr Phos
lung and bronchial troubles, with; also patient is depressed, languid and weak....Kali Phos
nervous, weak, tearful, anemic females....Kali Phos
sharp pains, with....Mag Phos
shock, mental, from....Kali Phos
tearful patients....Kali Phos, Nat Mur

## ANEMIA

blood is thin and watery; feeling of coldness in back; skin is dirty and sallow-looking especially in young girls, frequent palpitations, melancholy, bad dreams, constipation, backache, and other symptoms such as chills, feverish episodes, perspiration, neuralgia, delayed menses; excellent remedy....Nat Mur
builds up new blood cells....Calc Phos, Ferr Phos
cerebral....Kali Phos
children, of....Calc Phos
ear trouble, with....Ferr Phos
eyes have blue rings under them, decreased red blood cells, lips

pale, tendency to cough, headache....Ferr Phos
girls, young, in....Calc Phos
heart troubles, with....Kali Phos
infants, in....Silica
menstruation, prolonged, due to....Calc Phos
nervousness, with....Kali Phos, Kali Sulph, Mag Phos
obstinate cases may do better with higher potencies of the indicated remedy....indicated remedy
profound changes, without; red blood cells and hemoglobin are deficient....Nat Mur
puberty; young girls with skin pallor, weight loss, fatigue, decreased appetite, feel cold, constipation, delayed or irregular menstrual period....Ferr Phos
simple....Calc Phos, Ferr Phos
skin appears waxy, headache, ringing in ears, vertigo, extremities cold, tendency to excessive flow during period; give Ferr Phos as soon as there are signs of improvement in general health....Calc Phos
skin eruptions, accompanied by....Kali Mur
spinal....Kali Phos, Nat Phos, Nat Mur
young, rapidly growing people, of....Calc Phos

## ANEURYSM
anxiety, accompanied by....Kali Phos
general, in....Calc Fluor, Ferr Phos

## ANGINA (should be treated by a Doctor)
false....Mag Phos
pectoris....Mag Phos, Kali Phos, Ferr Phos

## ANKLES (see also Extremities)
feel as if dislocated....Calc Phos
pain in....Nat Mur, Silica, Ferr Phos
weak....Silica, Nat Phos, Nat Mur

## ANTACID, major remedy for digestion....Nat Phos

## ANTIBIOTIC, children, especially with fever, congestion, and coughing....Ferr Phos

## ANTI-INFECTION....Silica

## ANTISEPTIC....Kali Phos

## ANTISPASMODIC, bowels, stomach, throat, larynx, corners of the

mouth are especially affected; primary remedy; also Calc Phos for spasms; supplements the action of Kali Phos....Mag Phos

ANUS (see also Rectum)

    abscess, painful....Calc Sulph
    cracks and fissures of....Calc Fluor
    fissures....Calc Fluor, Silica, Calc Phos, Nat Mur
    fistulas
        general, in....Calc Sulph, Calc Fluor, Silica, Calc Phos
        odor of sulphur....Kali Sulph
    herpetic eruption around area....Nat Mur
    itching
        aggravated at night....Nat Phos
        general, in; eliminate all citrus juice....Calc Phos, Calc
            Fluor, Nat Phos, Kali Sulph, Nat Sulph
    neuralgia of....Calc Phos
    pain in....Kali Mur
    prolapse....Calc Sulph, Kali Phos, Nat Mur
    rawness....Nat Phos
    soreness....Nat Phos, Nat Mur
    sphincter control, loss of....Calc Phos
    tendency to prolapse....Ferr Phos
    wart-like eruptions on....Nat Sulph

APPENDICITIS....dissolve in hot water and taken in frequent sips; in an hour repeat. Decrease frequency with improved symptoms....Ferr Phos, Kali Mur, Mag Phos

APPETITE

    abnormal, and food causes distress....Calc Phos
    curbing, helps, especially before dinner....Calc Fluor, Calc Phos
    decreased....Kali Phos
    excessive....Nat Mur, Kali Phos, Silica, Calc Phos
    hungry
        feeling of....Kali Phos
        ravenous....Nat Mur
        soon after eating....Kali Phos
        very....Silica
    increased....Calc Phos, Calc Sulph, Kali Phos, Nat Mur, Silica
    loss of, with flatulence, and acidity; especially good after any
        acute illness or when there has been any drain on the system....Calc Phos
    nervous weakness, associated with, and an empty feeling in

abdomen....Kali Phos

not satisfied....Kali Phos

poor....Nat Phos, Nat Sulph, Calc Phos

sudden, ravenous....Calc Sulph, Nat Mur

## APTHOUS ULCERS (see Mouth, Ulcers)

## ARMS (see also Extremities)

heavy feeling....Silica

tired....Nat Phos

## ARTERIES (see Blood Vessels)

ARTERIOSCLEROSIS....Nat Phos, Silica, Nat Sulph, Calc Fluor, Ferr
Phos, Silica

## ARTHRITIS

acute

gout, with; in chronic cases give Nat Sulph alone (see
also Gout)....Ferr Phos, Nat Sulph

swelling; white coating on the tongue; worse movement....Kali Mur, Ferr Phos

chronic; joints crack, synovitis, gout....Nat Mur, Nat Phos, Silica

fever symptoms are present, when; this remedy may be used as an
intercurrent remedy later in the disease....Ferr Phos

general, in; results have proven better when salts have been dissolved in some hot water and taken in sips....Nat Phos, Ferr
Phos, Kali Mur, Calc Fluor, Silica

inflammation, with....Ferr Phos

joints, deposits in (see also Joints, Gout)....Silica

pain, violent and spasmodic....Mag Phos

suppuration of joints

general, in....Silica

process, in....Calc Sulph

violent pains, with; useful as an intercurrent remedy for violent
pains; pain is excruciating and spasmodic....Mag Phos

## ARTHRITIS, RHEUMATIC

enlargements, gouty, of the finger joints (see also Gout)....Calc
Fluor

finger joints, especially; urine red; pains go suddenly to the heart;
sore hamstrings; helpful in hot painful swellings of knee
joints....Nat Mur, Nat Sulph

gout, with; worse at night and during bad weather....Calc Phos

joints, in (see Joints)
pain (see also Pain)
>joints, in, with cold or numb feeling; worse cold and
from change of weather....Calc Phos
shifts from one joint to another; worse heat....Kali Sulph

ARTICULATION (see Speech)

ASPHYXIA, dissolve six tablets of each together in hot water and give in
frequent sips....Kali Phos, Nat Mur, Ferr Phos

ASSIMILATION (see Digestion, Stomach)

ASTHMA
aggravates symptoms
air heated....Kali Sulph
atmosphere dusty....Silica
food, any....Kali Phos
weather
damp, change to....Nat Sulph
warm....Kali Sulph
wet....Nat Sulph
allergic origin or neurogenic....Kali Phos
anemia, with; give with any other indicated remedy....Calc Phos
awakens at night with attack....Nat Sulph
bilious....Nat Sulph, Kali Mur
breathing labored; give frequently....Kali Phos
bronchial
catarrh, with; worse in warm season (see also
Catarrh)....Kali Sulph
lungs filled with loose, yellowish or greenish matter that
is easily coughed; up; worse evenings, humid conditions, and hot, stuffy atmosphere; copious expectorate....Kali Sulph
recurrent, helps to prevent; accompanied with clear,
gluey and tough expectorate (see also Expectoration)
....Calc Phos
yellow sputum, with....Calc Phos
cardiac asthma....Kali Phos, Kali Mur
children, especially, who suffer attacks after some skin disease,
such as eczema, or suppression of skin problems; wheezes at
every change in the weather; give Nat Sulph 12X for a few
weeks then give Calc Phos 3X....Nat Sulph

cough (see Cough)

expectoration (see Expectoration)

flatulence, with....Mag Phos

gasping and tightness, with....Mag Phos, Nat Sulph

gastric derangements, with....Kali Mur, Nat Sulph

humid

> general, in....Nat Sulph
>
> rattling, coarse, with increased chest congestion, mucus, and sweating feet....Silica

mucus (see Discharge, Expectoration)

nervous; helps breathing; worse mental and physical exertion or cold; better rest, warmth, and sometimes eating....Mag Phos, Kali Phos

phlegm is thick, tenacious, greenish-yellow....Nat Sulph

primary remedy for asthma; hard, asthmatic cough with thick expectoration and a constant desire to take long, deep breaths, especially if aggravated by wet, warm weather; good combined with Silica....Nat Sulph

salivation, with....Nat Mur

spasmodic, nervous....Mag Phos, Kali Phos

stomach or bowel upsets, with....Kali Mur

wheezing, nausea and loose cough, with; alternate with Mag Phos every 1/4 to 1/2 hour....Ferr Phos

ATROPHY, treating the cause is important....Calc Phos, Silica, Kali Mur, Kali Phos

AUTOINTOXICATION, removes poison charged fluids....Nat Sulph

AUTOTOXEMIA (see also Cleanser, Sepsis)....Nat Phos, Kali Phos, Kali Mur

AVERSION TO

> acid-type foods....Mag Phos
>
> alcohol....Silica
>
> bread....Nat Mur
>
> coffee....Calc Sulph, Mag Phos, Ferr Phos
>
> fatty food....Nat Phos, Kali Mur
>
> foods normally liked....Nat Phos
>
> herring....Ferr Phos
>
> hot drinks....Kali Sulph
>
> meat....Silica, Calc Sulph, Ferr Phos
>
> milk....Ferr Phos

salty food....Nat Mur
sour food....Ferr Phos
sweets....Kali Phos
warm food....Silica
work....Silica

AWAKENED
> flatulent pains, by....Nat Sulph
> screaming....Kali Phos

AWKWARDNESS....Mag Phos

AXILLA, perspiration (see Perspiration)

BACK
> ache
>> acute inflammatory pains; give Kali Mur if other indicated remedies do not cure....Ferr Phos
>> aggravates condition
>>> evening....Kali Sulph
>>> lying on something hard....Nat Mur
>>> motion, by....Silica
>>> warm room....Kali Sulph
>> ameliorates (makes symptoms better)
>>> lying on something hard....Nat Mur
>>> motion, by....Calc Fluor
>>> open air, in....Kali Sulph
>> dragging sensation, with; pain or fatigue accompanied by a full feeling and confined bowels; take every 1/2 hour; sponge area with mixture of 1-2 tablets in a small glass of water....Calc Fluor
>> general, in; precede with Ferr Phos....Calc Phos
>> lumbar region on arising in morning....Calc Phos
>> menstrual periods, with; alternate with Ferr Phos....Kali Mur, Ferr Phos
>> growing pains in young people with backaches, and after exertion....Calc Phos
>> lower back pains
>>> bearing down pains; tired feeling....Calc Fluor, Ferr Phos, Nat Mur
>> morning, in, with numbness, coldness and creeping sensation in the small of the back....Calc Phos
>> nape, extends to....Silica

neuralgic pains, boring, darting....Mag Phos
obstinate....Calc Fluor
scapulas, between....Kali Phos, Calc Phos
severe....Calc Fluor, Nat Mur
shoulders, of....Calc Phos
soreness up and down spine....Nat Sulph
uterine pain, with....Calc Phos
asleep....Calc Phos
cold....Nat Mur, Calc Phos, Silica
coldness feeling in....Nat Mur
crick in....Ferr Phos, Calc Sulph
dragging sensation in small of back....Calc Fluor
lame....Nat Mur
numbness and weakness....Kali Phos
pain
    acute, boring....Mag Phos
    bearing down pains in the lower back with a tired feel-ing....Calc Fluor, Ferr Phos, Nat Mur
    darting....Mag Phos
    general, in; add Nat Sulph, Nat Phos, Kali Phos if the following remedies don't work; precede with Ferr Phos....Calc Phos, Calc Fluor, Nat Mur
    inflammatory over kidneys....Ferr Phos
    low back (see Back, ache)
    motion relieves....Kali Phos
    neuralgic
        boring, darting pain....Mag Phos
        general, in....Kali Sulph, Mag Phos
    rheumatic, wandering, shifting....Kali Sulph
    sacro-iliac synchondrosis, with pain....Calc Phos
    sacrum
        lower....Calc Phos
        stool, after....Calc Phos
    scapulas, between....Calc Phos, Kali Phos
    shoulders
        aching of....Calc Phos
        soreness between....Silica
    spasmodic....Silica, Mag Phos
soreness up and down spine....Nat Sulph
spasms in....Nat Sulph, Mag Phos, Calc Phos
stiff; motion makes symptoms worse....Ferr Phos

tingling sensation....Mag Phos
weak feeling in....Nat Phos

BACKWARDNESS, where there is bone weakness or recurring tooth troubles....Calc Fluor

BALANITIS (see Sexual Organs, Male)

BALDNESS (see Alopecia)

BED SORES, these remedies can be applied locally in a compress (see also Ulcerations)....Kali Phos, Ferr Phos

BED WETTING (see also Enuresis)
children, when other remedies fail....Kali Phos
general, in....Calc Phos, Ferr Phos
liquids, increased, before bed....Nat Phos
worms, caused by....Ferr Phos, Kali Phos, Calc Phos, Silica

BELCHING (see Eructations)

BILE
excessive....Nat Sulph
lack of....Kali Mur

BILIOUSNESS (see also Liver)
acidity, with....Nat Phos, Nat Sulph
ailments of the liver, with....Nat Sulph
bile, from too much....Nat Sulph
bilious fever; dissolve 3 of each in hot water and take in frequent
    sips; repeat as often as necessary....Nat Phos, Nat Sulph, Ferr
    Phos, Nat Mur
colic, with....Nat Sulph
fever, with....Nat Phos, Mag Phos, Nat Sulph
general, in....Nat Sulph, Calc Sulph
irritability, with....Nat Sulph
notably....Nat Sulph, Calc Sulph
rich foods cause....Kali Mur
tongue (see also Tongue, coating)
        bright yellow fur coating, associated with....Nat Phos
        white/gray coating, associated with; may have sallow
            skin, yellow eyeballs, liver region sore,
            flatulence....Nat Sulph, Kali Mur

BITES AND STINGS of insects; dissolve 5 of each in hot water; take in frequent sips; increase the solution and apply locally as a compress....Nat Mur, Nat Phos, Kali Phos

BLADDER DISORDERS (see also Urine)
> can't hold urine....Ferr Phos, Nat Phos
> catarrh....Nat Mur, Kali Mur, Calc Sulph
> constant urge to urinate
>> chronic....Kali Mur, Silica
>> general, in....Mag Phos, Calc Phos, Nat Phos, Nat Sulph
>> if not chronic....Ferr Phos
>> standing or walking; spasmodic retention of urine....Mag Phos
> cutting pain
>> neck of bladder, in....Calc Phos, Kali Phos, Ferr Phos
>> urination, after....Nat Mur, Calc Phos, Kali Phos
> cystitis (see Cystitis)
> debility of bladder....Nat Phos
> desire to urinate, with scanty emission....Silica
> dysuria with slow start of flow; cutting/burning sensation in urethra or bladder when voiding; rule out prostate problems....Nat Mur
> inflammation....Kali Mur, Ferr Phos, Calc Sulph
> irritation at neck of bladder....Ferr Phos
> paralysis, due to nervous origin....Kali Phos
> smarting on urination....Ferr Phos
> spasms of bladder
>> general, in....Mag Phos
>> painful straining, with....Mag Phos, Kali Phos, Ferr Phos
> sphincter control, loss of....Calc Phos
> spurts out urine during coughing....Ferr Phos, Nat Mur
> stones, with....Calc Phos, Silica, Mag Phos, Nat Sulph
> suppression, urinary....Ferr Phos
> urethra problems (see Urethra)
> urge, frequently....Mag Phos, Ferr Phos, Nat Phos, Calc Phos, Nat Sulph
> weakness with frequent urination....Calc Phos

BLEEDING into the tissues (see also Bruising); apply powder directly to area....Ferr Phos

BLEPHARITIS with yellow crust formation....Kali Sulph

## BLISTERS

clear, watery contents....Nat Mur

fever blister on lips....Nat Mur

fingers, festers on....Nat Mur

fetid, watery contents, with....Kali Phos

general, in; give 5 of each dissolved in tepid water and apply topically as a compress....Nat Mur, Kali Phos, Ferr Phos, Kali Mur,
Nat Sulph

painful, and blebs on the skin, with watery contents....Nat Mur

pearl-like, at corners of mouth....Nat Mur

skin, on; also apply topically to burns and scalds; give Ferr Phos
to relieve the pain....Kali Mur, Kali Phos, Nat Mur

tongue, tip of....Nat Phos, Nat Sulph, Nat Mur

watery; chief remedy....Nat Mur

## BLOATED....Nat Mur

## BLOOD

acid condition of the blood, ailments arising from; reduces acidity....Nat Phos

alkaline, helps to remain....Mag Phos

anemia; thin, watery blood (see also Anemia)....Nat Mur, Calc
Phos

cells (see Red Blood Cells)

coagulating, not....Kali Phos

dark....Kali Phos

formation of red blood, helps in....Ferr Phos

healer and purifier....Calc Sulph

impurities, for conditions that arise from....Calc Sulph

oxygen to be carried by the blood to all cells, helps....Ferr Phos,
Kali Sulph

primary first aid remedy because it carries oxygen throughout the
body and strengthens the walls of the blood vessels, especially
arteries....Ferr Phos

purifier, systemic....Calc Sulph, Kali Mur

rushes to the head....Ferr Phos, Nat Sulph

thickened, forms clots....Kali Mur

thin....Kali Phos

thin and watery with pallor of the skin, depression and prostration; skin may sometimes be greasy....Calc Phos, Nat Mur

## BLOOD CELLS, to increase....Calc Phos

BLOOD POISONING....Kali Phos, Mag Phos, Nat Phos

BLOOD PRESSURE

> emotional causes, from (see also Mental States)....Kali Phos, Nat Mur
>
> high....Calc Fluor, Ferr Phos, Silica
>
> high, where there is no organ involved and nothing mechanical can be found as a contributing cause....Kali Phos
>
> low (treat as for Anemia)

BLOOD VESSELS

> chief remedy; restores elasticity....Calc Fluor
>
> dilation of....Ferr Phos, Calc Fluor, Nat Mur
>
> diseased....Calc Fluor
>
> enlargement....Calc Fluor, Silica
>
> inflammation of....Ferr Phos
>
> strength and toughness, gives, especially arteries....Ferr Phos
>
> tumor of....Calc Fluor
>
> veins (see Veins)

BLOWS

> cuts, bruises, causing swelling....Kali Mur
>
> effects of....Kali Mur, Ferr Phos

BLUES, SUGAR; feel run down, sluggish; avoid sugar....Kali Mur

BOILS (also treat as for Abscess)

> beginning stage....Ferr Phos
>
> edges of nostrils, on....Silica
>
> external ear, around....Silica
>
> general, in....Calc Sulph, Kali Mur, Silica, Ferr Phos, Mag Phos
>
> pus formation, for....Silica
>
> tendency to, especially in springtime....Silica
>
> topically applied....Kali Mur

BONES

> bone weakness or recurring dental troubles....Calc Fluor
>
> brittle and thin....Calc Phos
>
> bruises on....Calc Fluor
>
> children's primary cell salt; head bones are slow in forming; for those who are slow in developing mentally, as well as physically....Calc Phos
>
> condyles swollen....Calc Phos
>
> deformities (exostosis, dental caries, spurs)....Calc Fluor, Calc Phos

disease

> any that are not the direct result of injuries; gives solidity to weak or soft bones....Calc Phos, Ferr Phos
> congenital....Calc Phos
> general, in....Ferr Phos, Silica
> nutrition, poor, from....Calc Phos
> surface of bones affected....Calc Fluor, Silica

exostosis on....Calc Phos, Calc Fluor

formation of, aids....Calc Phos

fractures (see Fractures)

growth of bones and teeth, for....Calc Phos

growth, in general....Calc Fluor

inflammation of the soft parts about the bone....Ferr Phos

involvement of bones....Calc Fluor

necrosis of....Silica

osteophytes....Ferr Phos

ostitis....Ferr Phos

pain

> deep seated; worse at night; better when movement of limbs....Calc Phos
> general, in....Nat Sulph, Calc Phos
> shin bone, of....Calc Phos, Nat Phos
> standing, worse....Calc Sulph

problems, all; major chemical constituent of bones....Calc Phos

rickets (see Rickets)

rough, uneven....Calc Fluor

skull, thin and soft....Calc Phos

suppuration of....Calc Fluor, Silica, Calc Sulph

teeth ailments, and....Calc Fluor

thin....Calc Phos

tumors of....Calc Fluor

ulceration of....Silica, Calc Fluor, Calc Sulph

## BOWELS

acid conditions of....Nat Phos

burning in....Silica

catarrh in....Kali Sulph

discharging mattery substance....Calc Sulph

dryness of....Nat Mur

heat in lower bowels....Nat Sulph, Ferr Phos

inactivity, abnormal; numbness....Nat Mur

looseness in....Calc Phos, Nat Sulph
lower end sore....Calc Fluor
neuralgia of....Mag Phos
pain in....Mag Phos, Nat Phos
paralytic conditions....Silica
protrusion of lining membrane....Kali Phos
sore and tender....Ferr Phos
spasmodic pains in....Mag Phos, Calc Phos
sulfurous odor of gas from (see also Flatulence)....Kali Sulph

BOWLEGS in children, with joint swelling....Calc Phos

BRAIN

chemistry of the brain, vital to....Kali Phos
children, troubles of....Mag Phos
concussion of (see Concussion)
fatigue

> fever....Kali Phos
> inflammation; first stage....Ferr Phos
> loose, feels as if....Nat Sulph
> mentally worn out....Nat Mur, Kali Phos, Silica
> pain, violent, at the base of brain....Nat Sulph, Nat Phos
> primary remedy for brain-fog in students; will restore sleep, appetite, confidence, and strength; give with Silica 12X; if there is a general coldness or a tendency to night sweats, then also give Calc Phos 6X before each meal....Kali Phos
> rush of blood suddenly to the brain causing dizziness, giddiness and sometimes delirium....Ferr Phos
> softening of....Kali Phos
> water in....Kali Phos

BREASTS

burning sensation in....Calc Phos
fistulous sinuses in....Calc Fluor
hardness of....Calc Fluor, Calc Phos
knots, kernels....Calc Fluor
lumps....Calc Fluor
mastitis-inflammation of the breast (see Mastitis)
pain in....Kali Phos, Mag Phos
tumors in....Calc Fluor

**BREATH**

> catch in....Ferr Phos
> fetid....Kali Phos, Nat Mur
> offensive....Nat Phos, Nat Sulph, Kali Phos, Nat Mur
> shortness of
>> exhaustion, with; worse motion, exertion....Kali Phos
>> general, in....Ferr Phos, Nat Mur, Kali Phos, Kali Sulph, Calc Phos
>> stairs, on going up....Kali Phos

**BREATHING**

> difficult, especially in damp weather....Nat Sulph
> harsh....Nat Sulph
> hurried, at the beginning of illness....Ferr Phos, Calc Fluor
> oppressed; give every 20 minutes or so during the attack....Kali Mur, Ferr Phos, Calc Fluor
> short....Ferr Phos, Kali Phos, Calc Phos, Kali Sulph, Nat Mur

**BRIGHT'S DISEASE**....Calc Phos, Kali Phos

**BRONCHITIS**

> acute states; better results if the salts are dissolved in hot water and taken in frequent sips....Kali Mur, Ferr Phos
> chronic....Nat Mur, Kali Mur, Ferr Phos, Silica
> evening, worse....Kali Sulph
> expectoration (see also Discharge, Expectoration, Catarrh)
>> slimy yellow....Kali Sulph
>> thick and lumpy; first treat with Ferr Phos, then the following....Calc Sulph, Silica
>> unpleasant, mixed with blood; first treat with Ferr Phos, then the following....Calc Sulph, Silica
>> watery and greenish-yellow; give every 2 hours....Kali Sulph, Nat Mur
>> yellowish....Kali Sulph, Ferr Phos
> first stage; give every 2 hours....Ferr Phos
> general, in; give Ferr Phos first for 24 hours; if loose cough, less pain and fever, alternate with Kali Mur every 2 hours; if loose cough and much rattling of mucus in the chest give with Kali Sulph every 2 hours....Ferr Phos
> inflammation and fever, give first for....Ferr Phos
> phlegm (see also Expectoration)
>> thick, tenacious, greenish-yellow....Nat Sulph

white, thick; tongue whitish/gray; stuffy feeling....Kali
Mur

second stage; thick white phlegm; give every 2 hours....Kali Mur

soreness, with heat and burning....Ferr Phos

## BRONCHI

catarrh of (see also Catarrh)....Nat Sulph, Kali Mur

congestion, with wheezing and rattling sounds....Kali Mur

inflammation of....Ferr Phos

## BRUISES

bleeding into the tissues, any; also apply powder directly to
area....Ferr Phos

bones, affecting....Calc Fluor

compress; dissolve 5 of each tablet and apply locally for the compress; take internally also....Ferr Phos, Kali Mur

cranial bones, with hard, rough, uneven lumps....Calc Fluor

feeling all over of being bruised....Kali Phos

hard, blue-black....Kali Mur

head, with pain....Ferr Phos

shock and after-effects of....Nat Sulph

suppuration, with (see also Suppuration)....Calc Sulph

swelling, with....Kali Mur, Ferr Phos

## BUNIONS

compress, hot; may be applied locally morning and night from
these salts; take internally also....Calc Fluor, Kali Mur

general, in....Silica

## BURNING SENSATION

breast, in....Calc Phos

chest, with soreness....Ferr Phos

ears....Nat Phos, Nat Mur

eyes, in....Ferr Phos

eyelids, edges of....Nat Sulph

face....Kali Phos

feet....Kali Phos

head, top of....Nat Sulph

kidneys, over....Ferr Phos

nettles, as from....Calc Phos

nose....Nat Sulph

pain, with....Ferr Phos

rectum....Nat Mur

soles....Calc Sulph, Kali Phos, Nat Mur, Nat Sulph
skin....Silica
stomach....Calc Phos, Ferr Phos, Calc Sulph, Kali Sulph
throat....Ferr Phos, Calc Phos
urination
    after....Nat Mur, Ferr Phos
    during....Nat Sulph
uterus, in....Nat Mur
vagina, after urination....Nat Mur

## BURNS

analgesic; dissolve 10-15 tablets of 3X or 6X in a small amount of water and apply as a wet dressing....Kali Mur
compress may be applied locally from these salts; renew every hour as needed; take internally also....Ferr Phos, Kali Mur, Kali Sulph
first aid treatment for first and second degree burns; apply the pulverized powder to the area....Kali Mur
sensation of burning....Calc Sulph
scalds, and....Ferr Phos
small area, on....Kali Mur, Calc Sulph
sunburn (see Sunburn)
suppuration (see also Suppuration)
    general, in....Calc Sulph
    promote, to....Silica

## BURSA....Calc Phos, Calc Fluor

## BURSITIS....Calc Phos, Silica, Calc Fluor

## BUZZING IN EARS (see also Ears, noises)

## CALCULI....Mag Phos, Calc Phos, Kali Mur

## CALVES, cramps in....Mag Phos, Calc Phos

## CANCER

epithelial....Kali Sulph
general, in....Kali Phos, Calc Phos, Kali Sulph, Calc Fluor, Silica
growths....Kali Sulph
pains of....Kali Phos

## CANKER SORES OF LIP AND/OR CHEEK

cracked at the corners....Nat Mur
gangrenous....Kali Phos, Silica

general, in....Nat Phos, Kali Mur, Kali Phos, Nat Mur

watery....Kali Phos, Nat Mur

**CARBUNCLE,** use also treatments under abscesses....Calc Sulph, Kali Mur, Kali Phos

**CARDIOVASCULAR (see also Heart)**

cardiac neuroses associated with tachycardia, palpitation, vertigo or faintness; spells brought on by mental or physical exertion or by emotional upset; remedy will not correct the mechanical problem....Kali Phos

**CATARACTS**

foot-sweat suppressed, after....Silica

major remedy; lens of the eye contains high concentrations ....Silica

progress prevented, especially when accompanied by right sided headache and eye pain....Calc Phos

pus, smoky, in anterior chamber....Calc Sulph

**CATARRH (see also Nose, Discharge, Secretion, Exudation)**

acidic; useful in all conditions....Nat Phos

acute; if catarrh is thick give Kali Mur instead of Nat Mur; give every 2 hours....Ferr Phos, Nat Mur

bronchial....Nat Sulph

chills and malaise, associated with....Ferr Phos

chronic condition; nose seems swollen or is ulcerated; patient takes cold very readily; give with other indicated remedies....Calc Phos, Kali Mur

clear, watery....Nat Mur

colds, with; watery, transparent frothy discharges....Nat Mur

conditions of; gargle or spray area....Nat Mur

coryza (see Coryza)

dryness and stiffness of nose; hawking of mucus from the back part of throat; after a week follow with Calc Phos....Kali Mur

early stage, with inflammation, throbbing, shooting pains....Ferr Phos

excessive....Nat Sulph

fever and congestion, with....Ferr Phos, Kali Mur

fever, with; give after Ferr Phos to promote perspiration....Kali Sulph

greenish....Calc Fluor, Kali Sulph

initial stages of, and inflammation; scarlet fever, measles, rheumatism, flu and all complaints associated with chills and malaise....Ferr Phos

loss of taste and smell, with....Nat Mur

obstinate cases where discharges are offensive, or where there is a painful chronic dryness of the nose, plugs in the nose, or ulceration of the mucous membranes; follow by Calc Fluor....Silica

old, with obstructed nose and loss of smell....Kali Sulph

raw egg whites, discharge looks like....Calc Phos

secondary stages associated with fevers and inflammations, with excessive formation of a thick, tenacious secretion; bronchitis, pleurisy with fibrinous effusion, croup, asthma, pertussis; presence of a white or gray coated tongue, with excessive secretions....Kali Mur

sinus, of (see Sinus)

slimy, yellow secretions....Kali Sulph

slow to respond to other treatments....Kali Sulph

sticky, yellowish secretions....Kali Sulph

stomach, of the....Kali Sulph

thick, lumpy, with pus-like secretions....Calc Sulph

third stage....Calc Sulph

watery, thin discharge....Nat Mur

white phlegm, thick, with stuffy feeling; chronic; difficulty breathing....Kali Mur

yellowish discharge....Kali Sulph

CELLULAR ACTIVITY; promotes healthy activity to the cells and restores tone to weakened organs and tissues....Calc Phos

CHANGE-OF-LIFE despondency....Kali Sulph

CHAPPED HANDS

cold, from....Ferr Phos, Calc Fluor

fissures of hands and feet, and, in which there is a thickened derma; persistent....Calc Fluor

CHAPS AND CHILBLAINS (see Frostbite)

CHEST

aching in....Calc Phos

colds; first remedy to use, especially in children....Ferr Phos

constriction of the chest; may be accompanied with throat constriction....Mag Phos, Nat Mur

contraction of....Calc Phos

heat in....Ferr Phos
holds chest while coughing....Nat Sulph
oppression....Mag Phos
pain

    across chest....Calc Sulph

    angina, false,....Mag Phos

    angina pectoris; should be treated by a Doctor....Mag
        Phos, Kali Phos, Ferr Phos

    best general remedies....Ferr Phos, Kali Phos

    darting....Nat Sulph, Mag Phos

    deep-seated....Silica

    heart, over....Mag Phos

    left side, piercing....Nat Sulph

    pressure and breathing, from....Nat Phos

    sharp....Mag Phos

    sternum, above....Calc Phos

    rattling

        general, in....Kali Mur, Nat Mur

        great....Kali Sulph

        mucus, excessive....Kali Mur, Nat Mur, Nat
          Sulph, Kali Sulph

    soreness

        burning, with....Ferr Phos

        general, in....Calc Phos, Ferr Phos

        muscles, intercostal....Nat Phos

        touch, to....Kali Phos, Calc Phos

pressure ameliorates pain....Nat Sulph
tightness, feeling of....Mag Phos
troubles, with cold feet....Calc Phos
weakness in....Silica

## CHICKEN POX

convalescence (see Convalescence)....Calc Phos
eruptive period, during; alternate with Ferr Phos....Kali Mur
fever; from onset until fever subsides....Ferr Phos
required, the only remedies; only a few doses are needed; 5 tablets
    of each in hot water and sip a teaspoon every hour....Ferr Phos,
    Kali Mur
scaling of the skin, for....Kali Sulph
watery pustules; dissolve 5 tablets of each in hot water and sip a
    teaspoon every hour....Ferr Phos, Kali Mur, Nat Mur

## CHILDREN

ailments of; one of the most frequently needed remedies in the treatment of children's ailments; give with Kali Mur....Ferr Phos

bow-legs, with joint swelling....Calc Phos

complaint of muscle pains, especially in the left side of the body; teeth often appear soft and teething is delayed; upper lips are often sore and painful as well as the tongue; they also have trouble with digestion and elimination; other symptoms may be a poor memory, bad temper and slow mental and physical development....Calc Phos

crossness in....Kali Phos

cry out during sleep....Calc Phos

crying and screaming (see also Crying)....Kali Phos

debility in (see also Debility)....Ferr Phos

development, mental and physical, appears slow....Calc Phos

diarrhea (see Diarrhea)

diseases such as measles, chicken pox (see also the particular disease); give with Ferr Phos....Kali Mur

disposition unhappy, with symptoms of fretfulness, ill-humor, bashfulness, laziness, timidity....Kali Phos

emaciation in neck....Nat Mur, Calc Phos

feverish; give one tablet every hour until fever is gone if under 2 years old; over 2 years give 2 tablets (also see Fevers)....Ferr Phos

flabby, emaciated, sickly, ailing, backwardness....Calc Phos

foramen ovale, non-closure of....Calc Phos, Silica

fretful and/or peevish....Calc Phos

grinding teeth during sleep....Nat Phos, Kali Phos

growing pains....Ferr Phos

growth, helps; normal development aided....Calc Phos

gums, swollen; no teeth yet fretful and feverish; give every 2 hours for acute conditions (see also Teething)....Calc Phos, Ferr Phos

head sweats....Silica, Calc Phos

ill-tempered....Kali Phos, Calc Phos

infant (see Infants)

mental faculties, helps sharpen; maintains contented disposition....Kali Phos

night terrors....Kali Phos

nose bleed (see also Nose, bleeding)....Ferr Phos

pale face when teething is difficult....Calc Phos, Silica

peevish....Calc Phos

primary cell salt for children....Calc Phos

rawness of skin....Nat Phos

screaming at night during sleep    Kali Phos, Nat Phos

skin, for; keeps it healthy during illness....Kali Sulph

sleepwalking....Kali Phos, Nat Mur, Silica

swelling, soft, ailments with, such as mumps; give with Ferr
    Phos....Kali Mur

teething (see Teething)

tempers bad....Calc Phos, Kali Phos

thin, delicate looking for their age....Calc Phos

throat, sore (see also Throat)....Calc Phos

thrush (see Thrush)

tonsillitis, swollen, red and quite large (see also Tonsillitis)....Calc
    Phos

worse with fresh air and damp weather....Calc Phos

## CHILL

back, up and down....Mag Phos

daily at 1 p.m......Ferr Phos

fever, with (see Fever)

morning until noon; may be preceded by intense heat, headache,
    thirst, sweat, languor, emaciation, sallow complexion or blisters
    on tongue....Nat Mur

shaking, begins in the feet....Calc Sulph

## CHILLINESS

back, hands and feet; sensations are generalized in these areas;
    rule out abnormal thyroid function....Nat Mur

beginning of fevers, at....Ferr Phos

dinner, after; around 7 PM....Mag Phos

extremities, in....Nat Mur

feeling of being....Calc Phos

general, in....Silica, Kali Sulph, Calc Phos, Kali Mur

sensation of, especially the back; watery saliva; full, heavy,
    headache; increased heat sensation elsewhere....Nat Mur

## CHIN, eruptions on (see also Eruptions, Pimples)....Nat Mur

## CHLOROTIC condition....Nat Mur, Calc Phos, Ferr Phos

## CHOKING, generally, or choking when swallowing....Mag Phos

CHOLERA....Nat Sulph, Nat Mur

CHOLECYSTITIS-inflammation of the Gallbladder....Nat Sulph

CHOREA (see also St. Vitus' Dance, Nerves)....Mag Phos

CHRONIC

ailments, especially if severe inflammation is involved....Kali Mur

diseases; one of the most profound remedies for chronic disease....Nat Mur

CIRCULATION

disorders, congestive stage of....Ferr Phos

hands and feet feel cold....Kali Sulph

imperfect; when there is a condition associated with the circulation....Calc Phos

lower limbs and hands feel cold, especially in bed at night....Nat Sulph

parts feel numb and cold....Calc Phos

poor....Calc Phos, Nat Mur, Kali Phos

sluggish....Kali Phos

CIRRHOSIS, hepatic (see also Liver)....Nat Sulph

CLAMMY, feeling of being....Calc Phos

CLEANSER

cleans out accumulated non-functional organic matter, causes infiltrated parts to discharge their contents readily, and throws off decaying organic matter so there will not be injury to the surrounding tissues....Calc Sulph

detergent, acts like, in the large intestine and alimentary canal....Kali Phos

detoxify; used as a short term anti-toxic treatment....Nat Mur

purifier throughout the system, and....Calc Sulph, Silica, Kali Mur

removes poison charged fluids....Nat Sulph

septic conditions of the body, for....Silica, Kali Phos

toxic conditions; anti-toxic cell salts....Kali Sulph, Nat Mur

unhealthy tissue, for....Calc Sulph

COCCYX, painful after riding....Silica, Calc Phos, Nat Sulph

COITUS (see Sexual Organs, Male)

## COLD

being cold especially up and down the spine (see also
Chilliness)....Mag Phos
desire to go out in....Calc Sulph
hands and lower limbs (see also Circulation)
head, feeling in....Calc Phos
tonic for....Ferr Phos, Kali Mur, Nat Mur

## COLDS

after a cold; use to build up system....Silica, Calc Phos
air passages, involving....Silica
anemic people, in....Calc Phos
begins sneezing....Nat Mur
catch easily; take one dose of each per day during the cold season
to prevent....Calc Phos, Ferr Phos, Nat Mur
chronic....Calc Fluor
constant, have, especially if discharge looks like raw egg
whites....Calc Phos
cough, with (see also Cough)....Kali Phos
decreases length of illness....Calc Sulph
discharge (see Discharge, Catarrh, Coryza, Nose, Expectoration)
clear, watery, transparent mucus with sneezing....Nat Mur
frequent, with coughs and respiratory troubles....Ferr
Phos, Kali Mur
mucus, yellow, slimy....Kali Sulph
raw egg whites, looks like....Calc Phos
thick, yellow, purulent and sometimes tinged with
blood....Calc Sulph
disposition to catching cold in anemic people....Nat Mur, Calc
Phos
early; give during the first stage....Calc Sulph
eruption, vesicular, with....Nat Mur
final stages....Silica, Calc Phos
first feeling of cold symptoms, at....Ferr Phos
frequent, with cough....Ferr Phos, Kali Mur
general, in; dissolve 6 tablets each in a glass of hot water and sip a
teaspoon every hour....Ferr Phos, Kali Mur, Nat Mur
head cold
discharge that is produced by bronchitis (also see
Discharge, Nose, Catarrh, Coryza, Expectoration)
....Calc Sulph

dry skin, with; to produce perspiration....Kali Sulph
first stage....Ferr Phos, Calc Sulph
general, in....Ferr Phos, Kali Sulph, Nat Mur
greenish mucus, with a stuffy sensation....Silica, Kali Sulph
stuffy feeling, with....Kali Mur, Calc Fluor, Nat Sulph
thick discharge, with....Calc Sulph
yellow, creamy discharge from nose, with itching....Nat
 Phos
heated atmosphere, worse; also give Kali Sulph every 3 hours; if
 there is no runny nose omit the Nat Mur....Ferr Phos, Kali
 Mur, Nat Mur
inflammatory or first stage of....Ferr Phos
onset of cold symptoms....Ferr Phos, Kali Mur, Nat Mur
phlegm, white, and with congestion....Kali Mur
predisposition to catching cold....Ferr Phos, Silica, Calc Phos
running, watery colds are frequent, with chilliness and discomfort; skin is dry; cold sores on lips; loss of smell and taste....Nat
 Mur
sneezing (see Sneezing)
stuffy....Calc Fluor, Kali Mur, Nat Sulph, Kali Sulph
vesicular eruptions around nose, with....Nat Mur
watery mucus and sneezing....Nat Mur

## COLD SORES

general, in....Calc Fluor, Kali Mur, Nat Mur
lips, on; small....Nat Mur, Calc Fluor
mouth, corners of....Calc Fluor

## COLIC

acidity, with....Nat Phos
ameliorated by warmth and rubbing....Mag Phos
begins in the right groin....Nat Sulph
belching
  bilious....Nat Sulph
  general, in....Mag Sulph
  no relief with....Mag Phos
children, in....Calc Phos, Mag Phos, Nat Phos
cramps, with....Mag Phos
eating, with every attempt at....Calc Phos
flatulent
  bend double; children have legs drawn up....Mag Phos
  3X, Kali Phos

bowels, in....Mag Phos, Nat Sulph, Kali Sulph

general, in....Nat Sulph, Nat Phos, Mag Phos, Kali Sulph

relieved by warmth and pressure....Mag Phos

groin, right, starts in; bilious colic with bitter taste in the mouth; flatulent complaints after confinement or during menses....Nat Sulph

lower abdomen, in....Kali Phos

menstrual colic....Mag Phos, Kali Phos, Ferr Phos

nervous, tearful women, of....Kali Phos, Mag Phos

pain; may radiated from umbilicus; give every 10 minutes in a small amount of hot water until pain is gone....Mag Phos

pain has colicky nature, caused by sudden change from hot to cold....Kali Sulph

sour smelling stools, with; vomiting....Nat Phos

worms, due to....Nat Phos, Silica

## COLITIS

acute....Ferr Phos, Kali Mur, Kali Phos

pain, with; add the following....Mag Phos, Calc Phos

## COLLAPSE; take six of each in a small amount of hot water and sip frequently....Kali Phos, Mag Phos, Nat Mur

## COMA (treat as for Collapse)

## COMPLEXION

blotched; comes and goes suddenly....Nat Phos

bluish....Nat Phos

clear, fresh complexion, for

general, in....Silica, Calc Sulph, Calc Phos, Kali Sulph

pimples with pus, give additional for....Kali Mur

dirty looking....Calc Phos

feverish....Ferr Phos

florid....Ferr Phos

flushes easily....Ferr Phos

freckles, diminishes....Calc Phos

greasy....Calc Phos, Nat Mur

greenish looking....Calc Phos

greenish-white....Calc Phos

jaundice (see also Jaundice)....Nat Sulph

leaden....Nat Mur

livid....Kali Phos

pale

    pallid, and....Ferr Phos, Calc Phos

    sickly, sallow, and....Kali Phos, Calc Phos

pallid, from lack of red blood cells....Ferr Phos

red....Nat Phos, Kali Phos, Ferr Phos

sallow....Kali Phos, Nat Mur, Nat Sulph, Calc Phos, Ferr Phos

sickly....Kali Phos, Calc Phos

sunken....Kali Phos

waxy....Calc Phos

yellow, sallow, or jaundiced face, due to biliousness....Nat Sulph

yellow, pasty; may need to take for a few months....Calc Sulph

yellowish....Calc Phos, Nat Sulph, Kali Phos

## CONCENTRATION

difficult....Silica, Kali Phos, Ferr Phos

inability to, with forgetfulness and dull feeling....Mag Phos, Calc Phos

## CONCUSSION, BRAIN (see also Trauma)

blow, effects of....Kali Mur, Ferr Phos

chronic effects of falls upon the head, for....Nat Sulph

derangements from a head injury....Nat Sulph

general, in; dissolve in hot water and give in frequent sips....Kali Phos, Mag Phos, Nat Sulph

hemoptysis after concussion or fall....Ferr Phos

injury due to falling, worse since; may need high homeopathic dose; helps with mental troubles associated with falls on or injuries to the head....Nat Sulph

sight, having trouble with, after cerebral concussion....Mag Phos

## CONDYLES, swollen....Calc Phos

## CONGESTION

general, in....Ferr Phos, Kali Mur, Nat Mur

## CONJUNCTIVITIS (see also Eyes)

burning and grittiness of the lids....Ferr Phos

chronic....Nat Sulph

discharge (see also Discharge, Exudation)

    creamy, yellow....Nat Phos

    greenish....Nat Sulph

    thick, yellow....Calc Sulph, Kali Sulph, Nat Phos

    white....Nat Mur

    yellow, creamy....Nat Phos

yellow....Kali Sulph, Nat Phos
granular....Nat Phos
lacrimation, itching and irritated eyelids, catarrhal....Nat Mur
primary remedy, especially with inflammation....Ferr Phos
purulent, severe, in newborn....Kali Sulph
pus, with   Kali Mur
vesicles or pustules, with....Calc Sulph

**CONNECTIVE TISSUE,** a constituent of almost all connective tissues;
diseases of body membranes....Calc Sulph

**CONSTIPATION** (see also Stool)
acid, if very....Nat Mur, Nat Sulph, Nat Phos
alternate bouts of diarrhea, with....Nat Phos, Nat Mur
bashful stool; chronic, especially hard and dry; rectum seems to
have lost power to expel....Silica
bowels
paralyzed, seem....Kali Phos
relaxed....Calc Fluor
chronic....Nat Phos, Nat Sulph
dark stools....Nat Sulph, Kali Phos
drowsiness, watery symptoms from eyes or mouth, with....Nat
Mur
dryness of the bowel when other parts are watery....Nat Mur
elderly; often accompanied by depression, vertigo and
headache....Calc Phos
extreme....Kali Phos
fissures, anal, caused by hard dry stools; may alternate with diarrhea....Nat Mur
general, in....Calc Sulph, Ferr Phos, Mag Phos
habitual....Kali Sulph
hard to expel stool....Silica
hard stools with blood, especially in the elderly; associated with
mental depression, vertigo headache....Calc Phos
headache, dull, heavy, with; profusion of tears or vomiting of
frothy mucus....Nat Mur
heat in bowel, with....Ferr Phos
hemorrhoids, with....Calc Fluor, Nat Mur
inability to expel stool....Calc Fluor
inactivity of bowels, from....Nat Mur
indigestion, with; tongue white coated; worse with rich
foods....Kali Mur

infants, of; spasmodic pain with each stool and much gas; general
remedy for constipation in infants....Mag Phos
light-colored stools....Kali Mur, Nat Mur, Nat Sulph
moisture, lack of, from....Nat Mur
obstinate....Kali Sulph, Nat Phos
smarting after stool....Nat Mur
softening, helps, especially hard, knotty stools....Kali Sulph
tongue (see Tongue, coating)
torn feeling, bleeding, smarting after stool; hard, dry and difficult
to pass; associated with hemorrhoids, headache, and back
ache....Nat Mur
weakness of intestine, with....Nat Mur

## CONVALESCENCE (see also Vitality)

acute disease, of, to build up new blood corpuscles....Calc Phos
blood cells, provides new....Calc Phos
fever, after it has broken; time of rebuilding health....Ferr Phos,
Kali Mur
oxygenizes the blood; alternate with Calc Phos....Ferr Phos
restorative power speeds recovery and replenishes the body's
reserves of strength; tones up the system....Calc Phos

## CONVULSIONS

children, teething....Ferr Phos, Calc Phos, Mag Phos
development, during....Calc Phos
general, in....Mag Phos, Calc Phos
puerperal....Mag Phos
stiffness, with....Mag Phos

## CORNEA (see Eyes)

## CORNS, dissolve a few tablets of each in a little hot water and apply as a
compress....Calc Fluor, Kali Mur

## CORYZA (see also Catarrh)

alternating dry and loose....Nat Mur, Mag Phos
chronic....Silica
clear watery....Nat Mur
dry....Nat Mur, Calc Fluor, Kali Mur
fluent....Nat Mur
yellow, slimy....Kali Sulph

## COUGHS

acute....Kali Mur, Ferr Phos

ameliorated by cool, open air....Kali Sulph

asthma, from; chief remedy....Kali Phos

barking....Kali Mur

chest is very sore; mucus is thick and yellowish; sensation of
emptiness in the chest....Nat Sulph

chest pain, causing,....Ferr Phos, Nat Mur

children, in

      general, in....Kali Mur

      sickly, with night sweats....Silica

      suffocative....Calc Phos

chronic cases where the cough can be exhaustive....Silica, Calc
Phos

cold drinks, from....Silica

colds, with, frequent, and respiratory troubles....Ferr Phos, Kali
Mur

convulsive fits of coughing....Mag Phos

croup (see Croup)

croupy, from exposure to a cold wind....Calc Sulph

dry

      hard, tickling; also give Ferr Phos every hour....Kali
        Mur, Nat Mur

      severe, with difficulty speaking....Mag Phos, Nat Mur

hoarse....Calc Fluor, Nat Mur, Kali Sulph

evening, worse....Kali Sulph

expectoration, with (see Expectoration)

hacking....Kali Phos, Calc Fluor

hard, dry

      fever and soreness, with....Ferr Phos, Kali Sulph

      general, in....Ferr Phos

harsh....Kali Mur

hawking

      constant; to clear throat....Calc Phos

      fowl, slimy mucus; constant....Nat Sulph

      frequently....Calc Phos

      mucus from posterior nares....Kali Phos

      offensive, cheesy lumps....Kali Mur

headache, with; may be bursting....Nat Mur

hectic fever....Calc Sulph

herpetic eruptions, with....Calc Sulph

hoarse (see also Hoarseness)....Kali Sulph

holds chest while coughing....Nat Sulph

irritating....Silica
loose, rattling,
    general, in....Kali Sulph, Nat Mur, Silica, Ferr Phos
    thin, watery sputum, with....Mag Phos, Nat Mur, Ferr
       Phos
loud, noisy cough; croupy hard cough; thick white expectoration....Kali Mur
loud from the stomach and short; acute; check for a white tongue....Kali Phos
lying down
    aggravates....Mag Phos, Calc Fluor, Silica
    better from....Calc Phos
mattery expectoration, with....Calc Sulph
morning, early, worse....Nat Sulph
mucus, yellow....Kali Sulph
nervous....Mag Phos
night sweats, with....Silica
nosebleed, produces....Nat Mur
painful; may be with fever....Ferr Phos
paroxysmal....Mag Phos
periodical....Nat Mur
rattling of mucus, with....Kali Sulph
short
    acute, painful, irritating....Ferr Phos, Calc Phos
    dry cough after colds, chest has a sore feeling in it; feverish; give at first sign of respiratory problems....Ferr
      Phos
    general, in....Kali Phos, Ferr Phos, Kali Mur, Nat Mur
    irritation, with....Calc Phos, Ferr Phos
smells badly, breath, when coughs....Silica
spasmodic
    acute....Kali Mur, Mag Phos
    any; painful and persistent; whooping cough; worse
      night and lying down; dry cough in nervous
      patient....Mag Phos
    primary remedy....Mag Phos
splitting, constant, of frothy mucus....Nat Sulph
suffocative cough; worse lying down; expectoration tough and
    stringy....Calc Phos
tears to stream, causes....Nat Mur
throat sore, with expectoration of little granules....Silica

tickling, with

> general, in....Silica, Ferr Phos, Calc Fluor, Mag Phos
>
> larynx, in....Calc Fluor
>
> lumps of thick mucus, with....Calc Fluor
>
> sternum, behind....Nat Mur
>
> throat, in....Calc Fluor
>
> trachea, in....Ferr Phos, Kali Phos, Silica

tuberculosis patients, of....Calc Phos

urine, emission of, involuntary....Ferr Phos, Nat Mur

warm room, worse in....Kali Sulph

whooping

> chief remedy....Mag Phos
>
> general, in; dissolve 6 tablets of each in a small amount of hot water and sip immediately following each attack; keep solution warm....Ferr Phos, Kali Sulph, Kali Phos, Mag Phos
>
> vomiting, with....Ferr Phos

## COXALGIA....Nat Mur

## CRACKED LIPS (see Lips)

## CRADLE CAP....Kali Sulph

## CRAMPS

acute attacks that are repeated; dissolve 5 tablets of each in hot water and sip frequently; repeat every 3 hours....Mag Phos, Calc Phos

calves, in....Mag Phos, Calc Phos

general, in....Mag Phos, Kali Sulph, Silica, Calc Phos

limbs, in....Mag Phos

pain, shooting, darting or spasmodic....Mag Phos

stomach....Mag Phos

writer's....Mag Phos, Calc Phos

violin players, of....Mag Phos, Calc Phos

## CRAVINGS (see also Desires)

bacon, salty....Calc Phos

eggs....Calc Phos

pickles....Calc Phos

salt and salty foods....Nat Mur

sweets....Silica

meat, salted and smoked....Calc Phos

CRAWLING SENSATION

ants, feels like....Calc Phos
skin, on....Kali Phos

CROUP (see also Cough)

exudation and swelling, for....Kali Mur
failure of other remedies, if....Calc Phos
fibrinous exudation, with....Kali Mur
general, in; give every 15 minutes from onset; adding Calc Phos,
    Kali Sulph, and Kali Phos may be helpful....Ferr Phos, Kali
    Mur, Calc Fluor
primary remedy....Calc Fluor
spasmodic

chief remedy....Kali Mur
windpipe, in; causes it to close....Mag Phos

CRYING

children, in (see Children)
convulsive sobbing....Mag Phos
easily....Kali Phos
infants, of, during teething period; will prevent many unpleasant,
    restless and crying spells (see also Teething)....Calc Phos
tendency to....Mag Phos

CURVATURE of the spine; difficult sitting up; helps with healing....Calc
Sulph, Calc Phos

CUTS

abrasions, and; topical application of powdered tablets applied
    directly to the injured parts....Ferr Phos
shock and after-effect of....Nat Sulph
slow to heal....Calc Sulph
suppuration, with (see also Suppuration)....Calc Sulph
swelling, with....Kali Mur, Ferr Phos
wounds, and; apply powdered tablets topically for pain (see also
    Wounds)....Ferr Phos

CYSTITIS (see also Bladder Disorders)

acute....Ferr Phos, Kali Mur
chronic....Kali Mur
debility, with....Kali Sulph, Kali Phos
general, in....Ferr Phos, Kali Mur, Nat Phos
suppurating....Calc Sulph

## CYSTS

general, in....Calc Phos, Silica, Calc Sulph
watery....Nat Mur

## DANDRUFF (treat as for Alopecia)

primary remedy....Kali Sulph
sticky, scaly, moist; often a dry and scaly lower lip....Kali Sulph
supplement with this remedy....Nat Mur

## DEAFNESS

catarrhal congestion; closed Eustachian tube; acute....Kali Mur, Ferr Phos
chronic inflammation of Eustachian tubes resulting in diminished auditory acuity....Kali Sulph, Ferr Phos
cold, from a; follow in a few days by Kali Mur and Nat Mur....Ferr Phos
difficulty hearing
   exhaustion of nervous system, accompanied by....Kali Phos
   inflammation, from....Ferr Phos
   thick, yellow discharge, with....Calc Sulph
discharge causes (see Discharge)
Eustachian tube
   closed....Ferr Phos, Kali Mur
   swollen....Kali Mur, Silica, Kali Sulph, Nat Mur
general, in....Ferr Phos, Kali Mur, Calc Sulph, Silica
heated room aggravates....Kali Sulph
inflammation, due to....Ferr Phos
nerve troubles, due to....Mag Phos
nervous causes, from....Kali Phos
quinine, from taking; take especially morning and night....Nat Mur

## DEBILITY (see also Vitality)

acute disease, after....Calc Phos
aged, where there is an inadequacy of sphincter control and dribbling of urine....Calc Phos
atrophy, for (see Atrophy)
childbearing, from frequent; prolonged suckling....Calc Phos
emaciated (see Emaciation)
hysterical....Nat Mur
nervous states (see Nerves, Mental States)

nervousness, associated with; also sleeplessness and weakness from the least exertion that effects the patient mentally and physically; depression and in a sensitive state....Kali Phos 3X

puberty age girls, when restless and nervous; slow development, circulation imperfect, ears and nose cold, headache from artificial light, menses may be too early with faint feeling in stomach, back may be sore....Calc Phos

tone, restores, to weakened organs and tissues....Calc Phos

wasting disease (see Wasting Disease)

weakness, general debility, with constant desire to lie down and rest....Ferr Phos, Nat Mur, Nat Phos

DENTAL TROUBLE (see Teeth)

DENTITION (see Teething)

DERMAL FISSURES or cracks; persistent....Calc Fluor

DERMATITIS (see also Skin)....Ferr Phos, Kali Sulph, Kali Mur, Silica

DERMATOSES, vesicular, papular, and pustular, that leads to exude a yellowish-greenish discharge....Kali Sulph

DESIRES (see also Cravings)

ale....Ferr Phos

alcohol....Ferr Phos

bacon....Calc Phos

bitter things....Nat Mur

Claret....Calc Sulph

cold, to go out into....Calc Sulph

cool air....Kali Sulph

drinks, cold....Calc Sulph

fruit....Calc Sulph

ham....Calc Phos

indigestible things....Calc Phos

liquids because of intense thirst....Calc Sulph

meat, smoked....Calc Sulph

salty foods....Calc Sulph, Nat Mur, Calc Phos

sex

    no desire....Nat Phos, Kali Phos

    increased....Kali Phos, Mag Phos, Nat Phos, Nat Mur

    excessive....Nat Phos

sleep

    constant....Nat Mur

    mornings, in....Kali Phos

smoking, for....Nat Mur
stimulants....Ferr Phos
sugar....Mag Phos
swallow, constant desire to....Kali Phos
sweet foods....Calc Sulph
tart or sour food....Calc Sulph
vegetables
    green....Calc Sulph
    sour....Calc Sulph

## DETOXIFY (see Cleanser)

## DEVELOPMENT, irregular....Calc Phos

## DIABETES

chief remedy....Nat Sulph
craves bacon or salt....Calc Phos
depressing emotions, after; patient is weak, nervous, and restless....Kali Phos
dry mouth, with....Calc Phos
first signs of....Nat Mur, Nat Phos, Mag Phos
mellitus, due to faulty glycogenosis and glycogenolysis....Nat Sulph
nervous disease, with....Kali Phos
thirst, great; much wasting and constipation....Nat Mur
weakness, with....Kali Mur

## DIARRHEA

acid, sour smelling and greenish in color; due to gastric and intestinal fermentation....Nat Phos
alternating with constipation....Nat Mur
bilious....Nat Sulph
bloody stools or much mucus; tongue coated white....Kali Mur
children, in
    bloody and dry, or whitish-yellow stool....Calc Sulph
    general, in....Ferr Phos
    green and sour smelling....Nat Phos
chill causes....Ferr Phos
chronic; give night, morning, and after every evacuation; give also Ferr Phos if weak or elderly ....Calc Phos, Nat Sulph
cold drinks, ice cream, fruit, caused by....Calc Phos
constipation alternates; Nat Mur may also be helpful....Nat Phos, Nat Sulph

cramps, with

> general, in....Mag Phos, Kali Phos
> watery stools, and....Mag Phos

dark stools, bilious....Nat Sulph

depression, with....Kali Phos

digestive disturbances, from....Calc Phos

emotional upset caused by fright, from....Kali Mur, Kali Phos

excoriating....Nat Mur

exhaustion, with....Kali Phos, Calc Phos

fatty, rich foods, or pastries, after....Kali Mur

flatulence, fetid, with....Calc Phos, Kali Phos

fright, from....Kali Phos, Kali Mur

frothy....Nat Mur

fruit, from....Calc Phos

general, in....Ferr Phos

greasy, fatty food, after eating....Kali Mur

greenish

> bilious stools, with, or vomiting of bile....Nat Sulph
> general, in....Nat Sulph, Nat Phos, Calc Phos

gushing stools, frequent....Calc Sulph, Ferr Phos, Calc Phos

infants, in....Silica, Calc Phos, Nat Phos

involuntary, watery....Kali Phos, Nat Mur

jaundice, with....Nat Phos

maple sugar, after eating....Calc Sulph

morning

> evening, and....Calc Sulph
> worse....Nat Sulph

mucus, passing

> blood stained....Ferr Phos
> much....Kali Mur
> yellow....Nat Phos, Kali Mur

nervous condition, associated with....Kali Mur

offensive; take after meals....Kali Phos

painless....Kali Phos

pains

> cramping and flatulence; to give additionally....Mag
>     Phos
> severe....Mag Phos

pale stools

> clay-colored, with swelling of abdomen....Kali Mur
> rich food causes....Kali Mur

purulent....Calc Sulph, Kali Sulph

putrid, foul evacuations; depression and exhaustion of the
nerves....Kali Phos

rice water, passing....Nat Sulph, Kali Phos, Nat Mur

school girls, of, with headache....Calc Phos

severe....Mag Phos

slimy

> greenish to light yellow, sticky, watery....Kali Sulph
>
> yellow, with colic; may be watery or purulent....Kali
> Sulph

sore rectum and bowel prolapse....Kali Phos

soreness and smarting caused by frothy, slimy stool....Nat Phos

sour smelling

> general, in....Nat Sulph
>
> greenish stools, and....Nat Phos

spasmodic; include remedy indicated by the color of the diarrhea....Mag Phos

stool, with....Nat Phos, Kali Mur

straining at stool or constant urging to stool; passing of jelly-like
mucus indicating acidity....Nat Phos

summer diarrhea, with gastric weakness....Nat Phos

teething children (see Teething)

tongue coated yellow or creamy at the back....Nat Phos

undigested food, with....Ferr Phos, Calc Phos

unripe fruit, from; give every hour until better....Nat Phos

vaccination, after....Silica, Kali Mur

water-like....Nat Mur

watery stools

> expelled with force; gripping pain in abdomen....Nat
> Mur
>
> undigested, or; colicky pain....Ferr Phos, Nat Mur

weather aggravates

> change of....Calc Sulph, Calc Phos
>
> wet, after....Nat Sulph, Calc Phos
>
> yellow, slimy, purulent matter....Kali Sulph
>
> yellowish, tends to be....Kali Sulph

## DIATHESIS....Silica, Calc Phos

## DIGESTION

> aids in....Calc Phos, Silica
>
> appetite is lacking (see also Appetite)....Kali Mur

assists digestion and assimilation....Calc Phos, Nat Phos
discomfort with....Kali Phos
dyspepsia (see Dyspepsia)
fats, of....Nat Phos
fatty or rich foods, worse with....Kali Mur
flatulence, with (see Flatulence)
flushes of heat from digestive causes....Nat Phos
hydrochloric acid production, helps in....Kali Mur, Nat Mur
malassimilation....Calc Phos, Kali Sulph
prevents malabsorption of nutritional elements....Silica, Nat Phos
proper functioning of digestive organs, important for....Nat Phos
tongue white-coated; light-colored stools; biliousness....Kali Mur

## DIPHTHERIA

first stage, with ulcerated throat....Ferr Phos
general, in; dissolve 10 tablets of each remedy in a cupful of hot
    water and give one teaspoonful every few minutes; give also
    Kali Phos every 3 hours....Ferr Phos, Kali Mur
membranous exudation in throat....Kali Mur
most cases of....Kali Mur

## DISCHARGES (see also Expectoration, Catarrh, Exudation)

acrid....Silica
albuminous....Calc Phos
blood tinged....Calc Sulph
clear
    general, in....Nat Mur
    watery, transparent mucus....Nat Mur
corroding....Silica
creamy yellow; yellowish or golden-yellow; all cases....Nat Phos
excoriating....Calc Phos, Nat Phos
fetid....Silica, Kali Phos
fetid, yellow; associated with third stage of inflammation....Kali
    Sulph
fibrinous, stringy....Kali Mur
fluent coryza....Nat Mur
greenish
    general, in....Calc Fluor, Kali Sulph
    watery, and....Calc Phos
gushing....Mag Phos
lumpy....Calc Fluor

lumpy and thick with a bad odor; discharge is hard to detach and
goes back into the throat; may be green or yellow....Calc Fluor
non-transparent....Kali Mur
offensive....Silica, Kali Phos, Calc Fluor
offensive, thick, yellow....Kali Phos
one-sided from nose....Calc Sulph
opaque, white....Kali Mur
profuse, watery....Nat Mur, Kali Sulph
prostatic fluid, of....Nat Mur
purulent (see also Pus)....Calc Sulph, Silica
raw egg whites, looks like....Calc Phos
salty taste, with....Nat Mur, Kali Phos
slimy
    general, in....Kali Sulph
    yellow, watery, greenish, and....Kali Sulph
sticky
    general, in....Kali Sulph
    greenish, thick....Calc Phos
    white, thick....Kali Mur
    yellowish, from the skin or mucous membranes....Kali
      Sulph
thick
    tenacious mucus that adheres to tissue....Calc Phos
    white, and....Kali Mur
    yellow, purulent and sometimes tinged with
      blood....Calc Sulph, Silica
    yellowish, that is not offensive....Calc Sulph
vaginal (see Leukorrhea)
watery....Nat Mur, Kali Sulph
watery, free; flows easily....Nat Mur
white....Kali Mur
white, thick, fibrinous; may be white-gray, tenacious secretion;
    anywhere in the body....Kali Mur
yellow, slimy mucus or matter....Kali Sulph
yellowish
    general, in....Nat Phos
    thick, with pus and blood....Calc Sulph

DISEASE of body membranes; constituent of almost all connective
    tissue....Calc Sulph

DIZZINESS

attacks, subject to....Ferr Phos, Kali Phos
congestion, from....Ferr Phos
heart action, weak, from....Kali Phos
gastric derangements, from....Nat Sulph
general, in....Ferr Phos, Nat Sulph, Mag Phos, Kali Phos
inability to think because of dizziness....Silica
meals, after....Calc Phos
nervous people who don't assimilate foods well....Calc Phos, Kali
    Phos
vertigo (see Vertigo)

DOUBLE VISION (see also Vision)....Nat Mur, Mag Phos, Kali Phos

DREAMS

anxious....Nat Sulph, Nat Mur, Ferr Phos
anxious or vivid after late night snacks; not being able to sleep
    comfortably....Nat Phos, Nat Mur, Ferr Phos, Nat Sulph
awakens screaming....Kali Phos
convulsions from fright of dreams....Calc Sulph
danger, sense of, with....Calc Fluor, Mag Phos
falling, of....Calc Phos
frequent
    exclamations during sleep, with....Silica
    general, in....Nat Sulph
fire, of....Kali Phos
ghosts, of....Kali Phos
intense, anxious....Nat Sulph
lascivious....Kali Phos
nightmares
    anxiety from....Nat Sulph
    bilious symptoms, with....Kali Sulph, Nat Sulph
places, scenes, that are new, of....Calc Fluor
robbers, of....Kali Phos, Nat Mur
sexual desires, abnormal....Kali Phos
sexual....Nat Phos
vivid....Kali Sulph, Calc Phos

DROOLING....Nat Mur

DROPSY

blood, loss of, from....Ferr Phos, Calc Phos
general, in....Silica, Nat Mur, Calc Phos

heart
    disease, from....Calc Fluor, Kali Mur
    weakness, from....Kali Mur
  obstruction of bile ducts, from....Kali Mur

DROWSINESS
  bilious symptoms, with....Nat Sulph
  feeling of....Mag Phos
  general, in....Nat Sulph, Nat Mur
  great....Silica
  muscular weakness, with....Nat Mur

**Drugs,** cold tar, for counteracting the bad side effects of; drugs such as aspirin....Calc Sulph, Mag Phos

DRYNESS
  excessive, in any part of the system....Nat Mur
  skin, of (see Skin)
  sodium chloride deficiency, primary indication of; also for an over-abundance of water....Nat Mur

DUODENAL
  catarrh....Kali Mur
  ulcer....Nat Mur, Nat Sulph, Kali Phos, Ferr Phos

DYSENTERY (treat as for Diarrhea)
  blood, with....Kali Phos
  fever, with....Ferr Phos
  general, in....Ferr Phos
  purulent....Calc Sulph
  slimy....Kali Mur
  pain, with....Mag Phos
  purging, with....Kali Mur
  spasmodic retention of urine, with....Mag Phos

DYSMENORRHEA
  back, in....Calc Phos
  bearing down, during menses....Calc Phos, Calc Fluor
  before menses....Mag Phos, Kali Mur, Ferr Phos
  bright, red flow; face flushed, pulse quickened; excessive flow....Ferr Phos
  coldness, icy, with....Silica
  congestion, with....Ferr Phos

flow problem
    early, too, or too profuse....Ferr Phos, Kali Phos, Mag
       Phos, Nat Mur
    general, in....Silica, Ferr Phos
frequent urge to urinate, with....Ferr Phos
icy coldness, with....Silica
labor-like pains, with
    before menses....Calc Phos, Mag Phos
    during menses....Calc Phos, Mag Phos
lumbar region, while sitting or walking....Kali Sulph
membranous discharge....Mag Phos
nervous, weak, tearful, anemic females....Kali Phos
ovarian pain....Ferr Phos
pain extending to the thigh....Calc Fluor
precedes the flow....Mag Phos
prevent, helps....Ferr Phos
rheumatic pain....Calc Phos
sharp pain, to relieve....Mag Phos
vomiting of undigested food, with....Ferr Phos

## DYSPEPSIA OR INDIGESTION (see also Gastric Disturbances)
acid
    deficiency of....Nat Mur
    general, in....Nat Phos, Calc Phos, Silica
alcohol consumption, from....Silica
all cases, nearly; helps break up the food and promotes healthy
    digestion; take after every meal....Calc Phos
antacid; major remedy for indigestion....Nat Phos
appetite, loss of, with....Ferr Phos, Nat Phos
belching
    gas, with flatulence....Mag Phos
    general, in....Mag Phos, Nat Phos, Silica
    tasteless, burning....Mag Phos
bitter taste in the mouth; vomiting of bitter fluids....Nat Sulph
burning sensation beginning 1-2 hours after each meal and con-
    tinuing for a long time; may need to combine with Nat
    Sulph....Nat Phos
chronic....Silica, Nat Phos
damp weather, during....Nat Sulph
digestion (see Digestion)
excitement, too much; from fright....Kali Phos
face is hot and flushed....Ferr Phos

fatty greasy foods, due to....Nat Phos

flatulence; best given by dissolving 8 tablets of each in a cup of
really hot water; sip frequently (see also Flatulence)....Mag
Phos, Calc Phos, Kali Mur

flushed face and throbbing pain in stomach....Ferr Phos

heartburn and chilliness, with....Silica

hungry feeling after eating, with....Kali Phos

nervous, empty feeling (also treat as for Neurasthenia)....Kali Phos

pain, with

    after eating

        general, in....Ferr Phos, Nat Sulph, Nat Phos

        watery symptoms, with....Nat Mur

    salivation, and....Nat Mur

pressure felt in stomach....Kali Sulph

prevents malabsorption of nutritional elements....Silica, Nat Phos

rich, fatty foods and pastries causes....Kali Mur

risings acid, with....Nat Phos

spasmodic....Mag Phos

starch and fatty foods, due to ingestion of; may be associated
with flatulence, headache....Nat Sulph

supplementary remedy; helpful....Silica

tongue coating (see also Tongue)

    greenish-brown or greenish-gray....Nat Sulph

    slimy golden-yellow; associated with colicky pains in the
stomach and a feeling of fullness....Kali Sulph

    whitish-gray, after eating rich food....Kali Mur

vomiting; note tongue coating....Nat Mur, Ferr Phos, Kali Mur

watery risings, with....Nat Mur, Nat Phos

DYSPHAGIA (see Throat)

DYSURIA (see Bladder Disorders)

EARS

    ache

        albuminous discharge, accompanied by....Calc Phos

        beating, throbbing pain....Ferr Phos

        bones around ear ache....Calc Phos

        burning pain, with....Ferr Phos

        catarrhal inflammation of the middle ear....Kali Mur

        children, especially with discharge; bones around the ear
ache; may be accompanied by swelling....Calc Phos,
Kali Sulph

cold air aggravates....Mag Phos
congestion and swelling, with....Kali Mur
damp weather aggravates....Nat Sulph
discharge (see also Discharge, Exudation)
>blood, may be mixed with....Calc Sulph
>excoriating....Calc Phos, Nat Phos
>general, in....Calc Phos, Calc Sulph
>mucus....Kali Mur
>yellow; catarrh of the ear; children's ear
>ache....Kali Sulph
Eustachian tube swelling, associated with....Kali Mur
general, in....Kali Mur
glands, and
>painful; tonsils may also be painful....Kali Mur
>swollen....Kali Mur, Calc Phos
humming in ears, with....Kali Phos
inflammation or fever, with....Kali Mur, Ferr Phos
lightning-like pain through ears....Nat Sulph, Mag Phos
nervous or spasmodic conditions, from....Mag Phos
pulsating....Ferr Phos
roaring, with dullness of hearing and watery symptoms....Nat Mur
sensation of something forcing its way out....Nat Sulph
sharp, stitching pain....Ferr Phos
throbbing pain....Ferr Phos
tongue (see also Tongue)
>gray or white furred....Kali Mur
>white....Kali Mur
washing in cold water aggravates symptoms....Mag Phos
weather, damp, aggravates....Nat Sulph
wet or cold exposure, after....Ferr Phos
anemic people, troubles in....Ferr Phos
atrophic....Kali Phos
auditory canal, swollen....Silica, Kali Mur
blood flow to ear excessive....Ferr Phos
boils around external ear....Silica
burning sensation....Nat Phos, Nat Mur
calcareous deposits on tympanic cavity....Calc Fluor
catarrh (see also Catarrh, Discharge, Exudation)
>deafness, causing....Kali Sulph

Eustachian tube, of....Kali Sulph, Nat Mur, Kali Mur, Silica

inflammation with throbbing, shooting pains; initial stage....Ferr Phos

tympanic cavity, of....Kali Sulph, Nat Mur, Kali Mur

cold feeling....Calc Phos

confusion in....Kali Phos

congestive stage, such as with otitis....Ferr Phos

deafness (see Deafness)

deposit, thin, outer ear covered with....Nat Phos

discharge (see Discharge, Catarrh, Exudation)

blood, mixed with....Kali Phos

bloody

purulent, and....Calc Sulph, Kali Phos

thick and yellow....Calc Sulph

bright yellow....Kali Phos

chronic....Kali Mur

creamy

outer ear, of....Nat Phos

yellow appearance with scabs....Nat Phos

dirty....Kali Phos

fetid or foul....Kali Phos, Silica

offensive....Silica, Kali Phos, Kali Sulph, Calc Fluor

pain, with no relief of....Ferr Phos

purulent....Calc Phos, Kali Sulph, Nat Mur, Kali Phos, Silica, Calc Sulph

pus-like, thick....Calc Sulph

thick

white or gray and moist; may have granulations....Kali Mur

yellow....Silica

watery, yellow....Kali Sulph

whitish....Kali Mur

dry, scaly epidermis....Kali Mur

excrescence closing the ear....Kali Sulph

external meatus

swollen....Silica, Kali Mur

walls atrophied....Kali Mur

glands swollen in the area of the ear....Kali Mur

granulations within ear....Kali Mur

hearing, dullness of
    general, in....Ferr Phos, Silica, Kali Phos, Nat Mur
    nerve troubles, from....Mag Phos
heat in....Ferr Phos
heat and burning of the ears, with gastric symptoms....Nat Phos
inflammation
    bathing, after....Silica
    external ear....Kali Mur, Ferr Phos, Silica
    first stage for pain and fever....Ferr Phos, Mag Phos
    loud noise aggravates, and....Silica
    middle ear....Kali Mur, Mag Phos, Ferr Phos
    purulent discharge, offensive....Kali Sulph, Silica, Calc
      Phos, Kali Phos
    redness and burning in external ear....Ferr Phos
    swelling, with....Silica, Ferr Phos
internal parts are dark red....Ferr Phos
itching....Kali Phos, Nat Mur, Nat Phos
mastoid (see Mastoid)
meatus closed by excrescence....Kali Sulph
middle ear
    catarrh, chronic....Kali Mur, Nat Mur, Kali Sulph
    earache....Kali Mur
    general, in....Calc Fluor, Ferr Phos
    infections....Calc Sulph
    inflammation....Kali Mur, Mag Phos, Ferr Phos
    suppuration; chronic....Ferr Phos, Calc Fluor, Calc
      Sulph, Kali Phos, Silica
    swelling....Kali Mur
noises
    asleep, falling, on....Kali Phos
    beating in the ears....Silica
    blood pressure conditions, due to....Ferr Phos
    blowing nose, from....Kali Mur
    buzzing
      general, in....Kali Phos, Mag Phos
      humming, with....Kali Phos
      nervous exhaustion, from....Kali Phos
    cracking on blowing nose, chewing, when swallow
      ing....Kali Mur, Nat Mur
    crackling....Kali Mur
    drives you crazy; even small noises make you want to

scream....Kali Phos
ears or head, in, with confusion....Kali Phos
general, in....Ferr Phos, Nat Mur, Kali Phos, Kali Mur
hammering....Kali Phos
head, in; dullness of hearing with nervous symptoms;
    hears noise when falling asleep....Kali Phos
hearing better in noise....Kali Mur, Nat Mur
humming, from nervous exhaustion; helps with the
    elderly....Kali Phos, Nat Mur
pulsations....Ferr Phos
ringing like bells....Nat Sulph
roaring nature; cracking sounds in ears while
    eating....Nat Mur, Silica
running water, like....Ferr Phos
sensitive, over....Silica, Kali Phos, Ferr Phos, Kali Mur
singing or tingling....Nat Mur
snapping....Kali Mur
startled from least noise....Kali Phos, Kali Mur
study, excessive, causing roaring and buzzing....Kali Phos
tinnitus, aurium....Ferr Phos, Nat Mur, Kali Phos, Nat
    Sulph, Kali Mur, Calc Fluor
    whizzing and ringing, decrease of hearing....Mag Phos
    worse from....Kali Phos
one ear red, hot, burning....Nat Phos
otitis-an inflammation condition of the ear
    congestive stage....Ferr Phos
    discharge, with (see also Discharge, Exudation)....Calc
        Sulph
    suppuration, chronic, of middle ear....Calc Fluor, Ferr
        Phos
    suppurative; general....Silica, Calc Sulph, Kali Phos
pain (see also Ear, ache)
    bones, in, around ear....Calc Phos
    burning....Ferr Phor
    cutting, in or under ear....Ferr Phos, Kali Sulph
    general, in....Ferr Phos, Mag Phos
    inflammatory....Ferr Phos
    mastoid process, below....Kali Sulph
    nervous....Mag Phos
    radiating....Ferr Phos

sharp

in ear....Ferr Phos, Mag Phos

under ear....Kali Sulph

stitching....Kali Sulph, Ferr Phos, Nat Mur, Nat Sulph

throbbing....Ferr Phos

pimples around ear....Calc Sulph

pulsations in ear....Ferr Phos

red, dark, of internal parts....Ferr Phos

rheumatic complaints....Calc Phos

scabs, with creamy, yellow discharge....Nat Phos

scaling of tympanum, moist....Kali Mur

scrofulous complaints in children....Calc Phos

sore and scabby outer ear....Nat Phos

soreness; external ear....Nat Phos

stuffy sensation in....Kali Mur

suppuration, chronic, of middle ear....Calc Fluor, Ferr Phos

swelling

burning, itching, with....Calc Phos

Eustachian tubes, of....Kali Mur, Silica

external ear....Kali Mur

general, in....Kali Mur, Ferr Phos, Nat Phos

glands around ears....Kali Mur

meatus....Silica

parotid gland, with stitching pain....Silica

tympanic cavity, of....Nat Mur, Silica

tension in....Ferr Phos

tympanic cavity

catarrh....Kali Mur, Nat Mur, Kali Sulph

swollen....Silica, Nat Mur

ulcerated....Kali Mur

tympanic membrane

calcareous deposits on....Calc Fluor

discharge, whitish....Kali Mur

granular....Kali Mur

inflammation....Kali Mur, Mag Phos, Ferr Phos

moist exfoliation of....Kali Mur

red, beefy, dark....Ferr Phos

retracted....Kali Mur

swelling....Nat Mur, Silica

thickened....Ferr Phos

ulcerated....Kali Phos

tinnitus (see Ears, noises)

tissues

        dried up....Kali Phos

        scaly....Kali Sulph, Kali Mur, Calc Phos, Nat Mur

ulceration

        general, in....Ferr Phos, Kali Phos, Calc Sulph, Silica

        low forms of....Kali Phos

## ECCHYMOSES....Kali Mur

## ECZEMA

acidity, symptoms of....Nat Phos

anemia, especially if associated with....Calc Phos

bends of joints and eyebrows, in....Nat Mur

burning sensations, with....Kali Sulph

desquamation, yellowish....Nat Sulph

discharge, yellowish....Kali Sulph

dry....Calc Sulph

ears, behind....Nat Mur

eyebrows, of....Nat Mur

exudation (see Exudation)

itching, creamy exudate, scaling....Nat Phos

joints, bends of....Nat Mur

margin of hairy scalp, on....Nat Mur

overly sensitive....Kali Phos

salt, excessive, from....Nat Mur

scabs, white....Calc Phos

scalp desquamation which may produce Alopecia areata, or there

    may be nodules or pustules....Silica

scaly; if the scales are fine give Nat Mur....Silica

secretions, yellow-greenish....Kali Sulph

squamous....Silica

suppressed, suddenly....Kali Sulph

thickened and hardened skin, especially in damp weather....Calc

    Fluor

varicose ailments, associated with....Calc Fluor

vaccination, after....Kali Mur

vesicles

        watery....Nat Sulph

        whitish....Kali Mur

wet....Kali Sulph

## EDEMA....Nat Sulph

ELASTICITY
> loss of, with a consequent relaxed condition of muscular tissue and supporting membranes; results in muscular weakness and bearing-down pains; used for symptoms such as a relaxed condition of veins and arteries, piles, sluggish circulation, tendency to cracks in the skin; worse humid conditions; better from massage and warmth....Calc Fluor

ELBOW (see also Extremities, Joints)
> pain, shooting....Calc Phos
> soreness in bend of....Nat Mur
> swollen in joint....Calc Fluor

ELDERLY (see Aging)

ELIMINATOR (see Cleanser)

EMACIATION
> general, in....Calc Phos, Kali Phos
> while living well....Nat Mur

EMBOLISM....Kali Mur, Ferr Phos, Calc Fluor

EMOTIONAL (see Mental states)

EMPYEMA....Silica, Calc Sulph

ENAMEL, deficient in teeth (see Teeth)

ENCHONDROMA....Silica

ENDOCARDITIS
> chronic....Calc Sulph, Calc Phos
> general, in....Ferr Phos, Kali Mur

ENDOCRINE DEFICIENCY....Kali Phos, Calc Phos, Silica

ENERGY (see Vitality)

ENERVATION, all conditions of....Kali Phos

ENLARGEMENTS, gouty (see also Gout)....Calc Fluor

ENTERALGIA....Mag Phos

ENTERITIS....Kali Phos, Ferr Phos

ENURESIS (see also Bed Wetting)
> children, in
>> acidity, with; catarrh of the bladder....Nat Phos

habit, due to....Nat Phos
liquids, increased, before bed....Nat Phos
muscle weakness, with....Ferr Phos
nervousness, due to....Kali Phos
diurnal....Ferr Phos
elderly, in, with frequent urging to urinate....Calc Phos
general, in....Calc Phos, Kali Phos, Nat Mur, Ferr Phos
muscular weakness, for; if inflammation is present....Ferr Phos
nervous debility, due to....Kali Phos
nocturnal....Kali Phos, Mag Phos
paralysis of sphincter....Kali Phos
sphincter relaxed, if; give Calc Fluor for loss of elasticity....Kali
    Phos, Calc Fluor
walking or coughing, while....Nat Mur
worms, due to....Nat Phos

EPIDEMICS, helps prevent infection....Ferr Phos, Kali Mur

EPIGLOTTIS (see Throat)

EPILEPSY (see also Spasms)
blood rush to head, from....Ferr Phos
fright, from....Kali Phos
general, in....Kali Mur
night, at....Silica
suppressed eruptions, after....Kali Mur, Calc Phos

EPISTAXIS (see Nosebleed)

ERUCTATIONS OR BELCHING
acid condition from excess lactic acid....Nat Phos
belching brings back taste of food....Ferr Phos
bitter....Kali Phos
burning....Mag Phos
gas, with flatulence....Mag Phos
dyspepsia, with (see Dyspepsia)
gaseous....Kali Phos
greasy....Ferr Phos
hot drinks, from....Kali Mur
sour....Kali Phos, Nat Phos, Calc Phos, Silica, Nat Sulph
tasteless....Mag Phos

ERUPTIONS
anemia, with....Kali Mur

all kinds of; dissolve in water and apply to skin with a cotton
    swab....Silica, Calc Sulph, Calc Phos
boils around external ear....Silica
burning, itching....Kali Sulph, Kali Phos
chin, on....Nat Mur
discharge (see also Discharge, Exudate)
        clear, watery....Nat Mur
        sticky, yellow, watery....Kali Sulph
        thick, yellow....Silica
dry, especially on margin of hair and bends of joints....Nat Mur
eruptive diseases; to aid desquamation....Kali Sulph
exudations (see Exudation)
facial, that contain albuminous fluid with yellow-white
    scabs....Calc Phos
festers easily....Silica, Calc Sulph
head, on (see Scalp)
herpes; tablets can be dissolved in water and applied directly with
    a cotton swab (see also Herpes)....Calc Sulph, Kali Sulph
herpetic, on face....Calc Sulph, Nat Mur
itching at nape of neck on hair margin....Nat Mur
margins of hair at nape, on....Nat Mur
menstrual problems, with....Kali Mur
miliary....Nat Mur
occiput, on; offensive....Silica
painful, red....Kali Sulph
pimples, small, red, run together, making the face look swollen;
    tablets can be dissolved in water and applied directly with a
    cotton swab (see also Pimples)....Kali Sulph
pus (see Pus)
receding suddenly....Kali Sulph
scaling, with....Kali Sulph
scalp, on, with itching (see also Scalp)....Nat Mur, Ferr Phos
scaly, arising from a moist face....Kali Sulph, Calc Phos
second stage, with swelling and discharge....Kali Mur
skin and scalp, with scaling....Kali Sulph
stomach problems, with....Kali Mur
suppression of rash, sudden, in hot and dry harsh skin....Kali
    Sulph
sycotic-chronic inflammation of hair follicles....Silica, Nat Mur,
    Nat Sulph
vesicles; thick white contents; apply topically with a cotton swab

by dissolving remedy in water (see also Vesicles)....Kali Mur
watery contents, with....Nat Mur
thick, white contents....Kali Mur

## ERYSIPELAS

blistering....Kali Sulph
deep-seated....Silica
occasional....Calc Fluor
swelling of the skin, with....Nat Sulph
smooth, red, and shining....Nat Sulph, Ferr Phos
subcutaneous tissue, inflammation of....Silica
vesicular....Kali Mur

## EXHAUSTION (see Fatigue, Vitality)

## EXPECTORATION (see also Discharge)

blood streaked, scanty....Ferr Phos
clear, transparent....Nat Mur
constant
    hawking, and....Calc Phos
    watery, frothy....Nat Mur
copious....Kali Sulph, Silica
creamy....Nat Phos
difficult to cough up....Kali Mur, Calc Phos, Nat Mur
fetid....Kali Phos, Calc Sulph, Kali Sulph
frothy....Kali Phos, Nat Mur
granular....Silica
greenish....Silica, Kali Sulph, Nat Sulph
loose....Silica, Kali Sulph, Nat Mur
lumpy....Calc Fluor
milky....Kali Mur
mucus
    with tiny, yellow lumps; excessive....Calc Fluor
    general, in....Calc Phos, Calc Fluor, Nat Mur
    salty tasting....Kali Phos, Nat Phos
    slips back and is swallowed....Kali Sulph
    tough, in throat....Kali Sulph
    watery, coughed or vomited up....Ferr Phos, Nat Mur
offensive
    cheesy lumps, with....Kali Mur
    general, in....Silica
profuse....Silica, Kali Sulph
purulent....Silica, Nat Sulph, Calc Sulph

pus-like, excessive....Silica
rattling....Silica, Nat Mur
ropy....Nat Sulph
salty....Kali Phos, Nat Mur, Nat Phos
scanty and blood streaked....Ferr Phos
serous....Kali Phos, Nat Mur
slips back....Kali Sulph
slimy; may be yellow, green....Kali Sulph
tenacious, thick, white phlegm; give after Ferr Phos....Kali Mur
thick
>general, in....Kali Phos, Nat Sulph, Silica, Kali Mur
>ropy, and....Nat Sulph
>tenacious, greenish-yellow....Nat Sulph
>white phlegm; tongue, children's cough....Kali Mur
>yellow-green, and; profuse....Silica
>yellow lumps, with....Calc Fluor, Silica
tough
>lumpy....Calc Fluor
>stringy....Calc Phos
viscid, whitish....Kali Mur
watery and greenish-yellow....Nat Mur, Kali Sulph
white
>general, in....Calc Phos, Kali Mur
>thick or grayish-white; tenacious....Kali Mur
yellow
>lumpy....Calc Fluor
>rattling of mucus in chest, with; worse warm room, evening....Silica
yellow-greenish....Kali Sulph
yellowish....Kali Phos, Calc Fluor, Kali Sulph, Silica, Calc Phos, Calc Sulph

EXTENSORS, CONTRACTIONS OF....Nat Phos

EXTREMITIES (see also the particular body part)
aching, especially if due to poor circulation....Calc Phos, Calc Fluor
asleep, sensation as if parts were....Calc Phos
chilly....Nat Mur
clammy feeling in hands and feet, with inability to sleep late in the morning....Calc Phos
cold, numb....Calc Phos

cold feeling in hands and feet....Kali Sulph, Nat Mur, Calc Phos
coldness in....Nat Mur, Calc Phos
cold weather aggravates....Calc Phos
contortions of....Mag Phos
cramping pain, periodic; if Mag Phos does not relieve....Kali
    Sulph
cramps in....Mag Phos
crawling and creeping sensation in....Calc Phos
eruptions, herpetic, all over....Calc Sulph
exhausted feeling in....Mag Phos
fall asleep....Nat Mur
feel cold during the day and hot at night....Nat Phos
fidgety feeling....Kali Phos
injuries are festering from neglect....Silica
itch (see also Itching)....Kali Mur
jerking....Mag Phos, Nat Mur
neuralgia
        general, in....Mag Phos, Kali Sulph
        muscular contractions, with....Mag Phos
numb
        cold, and....Calc Phos
        general, in—-Nat Mur, Calc Phos, Kali Phos
pains, rheumatic (infectious) and gouty arthritis (see also
    Arthritis, rheumatic)
        circulation poor, due to....Calc Fluor, Calc Phos
        coldness and numbness of limbs, with....Calc Phos
        lameness, with....Ferr Phos
        motion aggravates....Ferr Phos
        neuralgia (see Extremities, neuralgia)
        shifting, settling in one place then another....Kali Sulph
        stiffness from cold, with....Ferr Phos
        tingling sensation....Mag Phos
        tired feeling, with....Silica
        trembling, with....Calc Phos
        twitching, with....Calc Phos
        weather changes, worse....Calc Phos
paralysis (see Paralytic Conditions)
sore, aching....Calc Phos
stimulants, worse....Mag Phos
swelling, hard....Calc Fluor
weather changes, worse....Calc Phos

EXUDATION (see also Discharge)
albuminous....Calc Phos, Nat Mur
bloody....Ferr Phos, Calc Fluor
causing soreness and chafing....Kali Phos, Nat Mur
clear....Nat Mur
creamy golden-yellow....Nat Phos
excoriating....Nat Phos, Calc Phos
fibrinous....Kali Mur
grayish-white....Kali Mur
green....Nat Sulph, Nat Phos
greenish, thin....Kali Sulph
hard and lumpy....Calc Fluor, Kali Mur
hardened....Calc Fluor
honey-colored....Nat Phos
irritating....Kali Phos
mattery or streaked with blood—-Calc Sulph
milky....Calc Phos
offensive....Silica, Kali Phos
painful....Calc Fluor, Mag Phos
purulent....Kali Sulph, Calc Sulph
ropy....Kali Mur
septic....Kali Phos
serous....Kali Sulph, Calc Phos, Nat Mur
soreness, causing....Nat Phos
sour odor or taste....Nat Phos
transparent, thin like water....Nat Mur
watery....Nat Mur, Nat Sulph, Kali Sulph
white and fibrinous....Kali Mur
yellow
   general, in....Nat Phos, Kali Mur, Kali Sulph, Nat Sulph
   gold-like....Nat Phos
   greenish-yellow, with thin crust loosely attached....Kali
    Sulph
   slimy....Kali Sulph
   smooth, tough lumps, with....Calc Fluor
   thick, pus....Silica

EYELIDS
   agglutination
    morning, creamy discharge....Nat Phos
    night; may have smarting type pain....Silica

boils around lids....Silica
burning
        edges....Nat Sulph
        general, in....Nat Mur, Kali Phos
crusts, yellow....Kali Sulph
cystic tumors, with....Silica, Ferr Phos
drooping....Kali Phos, Mag Phos
eruptions, crusted, yellow....Kali Sulph
grains of sand are under lids, sensation of....Ferr Phos
granulations
        general, in....Nat Mur
        lids, on....Ferr Phos, Kali Mur
inflamed....Nat Mur
irritated....Nat Mur
matter on eyelids, specks of....Kali Mur
spasm....Calc Phos, Mag Phos
styes (see Styes)
swollen....Kali Sulph
tumors of....Calc Fluor
twitching
        convulsive....Mag Phos
        general, in....Calc Phos, Mag Phos, Kali Phos
yellow with mattery scales....Kali Mur

## EYES

ache of eyeballs....Calc Fluor, Calc Phos
affections, with flow of tears....Nat Mur
ameliorates symptoms after closing and pressing lightly....Calc
    Fluor
asthenopia, muscular....Nat Mur, Mag Phos, Kali Phos
black spots before eyes....Kali Phos, Silica
blepharitis....Nat Mur, Silica
bloodshot....Nat Mur, Ferr Phos, Nat Phos
blurring (see also Vision)....Kali Phos, Calc Fluor
burning sensation in....Ferr Phos
canthi inflamed....Calc Sulph
cataracts (see Cataracts)
children, school, troubles in....Calc Phos
colors before eyes (see Vision)
color vision, abnormal....Mag Phos
concussion, trouble with their sight after (see also

Concussion)....Mag Phos
conjunctiva
    inflammation of (see also Conjunctivitis)....Kali Sulph
    ophthalmia-severe inflammation
        creamy discharge, with....Nat Phos
        thick and yellow discharge....Calc Sulph
    reddened or yellow....Nat Mur, Nat Sulph
    vesicular formations on epithelium....Nat Phos
    yellow....Nat Sulph
conjunctivitis (see Conjunctivitis)
cornea
    abscess; if in first stage also give Ferr Phos....Calc Sulph,
        Silica, Kali Sulph, Kali Mur
    blisters on....Nat Mur, Kali Mur
    flat....Kali Mur
    inflamed, with abscess....Calc Sulph, Ferr Phos
    injury....Calc Sulph
    keratitis-inflammation of cornea
        parenchymatous....Calc Phos, Kali Mur
        pustular....Silica, Calc Sulph
    opaque....Calc Phos, Silica
    scrofulous....Calc Phos, Nat Mur
    smoky....Calc Sulph
    spots on....Calc Fluor, Nat Sulph
    thick, yellow discharge....Calc  Sulph
    ulcer
        deep....Calc Sulph, Calc Phos
        edges hard, with....Calc Fluor
        flat....Kali Mur
        general, in....Silica, Kali Mur
        pus in anterior chamber behind cornea....Calc
        Sulph, Silica, Kali Mur, Kali Sulph,
        Nat Phos
    vesicular formations on the epithelium....Nat Phos
    white spots on....Nat Mur
crusts, yellow....Kali Sulph
discharge (see also Discharge, Exudations)
    clear, watery mucus....Nat Mur
    creamy, golden-yellow....Nat Phos
    golden, creamy....Nat Phos
    green pus....Nat Sulph

greenish; serous....Kali Mur, Kali Sulph
mucus
> clear....Nat Mur
> general, in....Kali Mur
> slimy secretions....Kali Sulph
> white,...Kali Mur

thick
> white....Kali Mur
> yellow....Silica, Calc Sulph

white....Kali Mur
whitish, with inflammation....Kali Mur, Ferr Phos
yellow-greenish....Kali Sulph, Kali Mur
eruption of small vesicles about eyes....Nat Mur
eyeball
> ache....Calc Fluor, Calc Phos
> pain in
>> motion aggravates....Ferr Phos
>> relieved by resting eyes....Calc Fluor
> soreness....Kali Phos
> yellowness....Nat Sulph

flickering before eyes....Calc Fluor
floaters; spots before eyes....Silica, Kali Phos
foreign body in, sensation of....Calc Sulph
general; take along with indicated remedy for eyes....Silica, Calc
Phos, Calc Sulph, Calc Fluor
glaucoma....Nat Mur
granulations, blister-like....Nat Sulph, Nat Phos
hemiopia....Calc Sulph
inflammation
> acute pain, with; great intolerance of light....Ferr Phos
> discharge of thick yellow matter, with....Calc Sulph,
>   Silica
> dry....Calc Phos, Nat Mur, Ferr Phos
> general, in....Ferr Phos, Calc Sulph, Calc Phos
> secretion
>> golden-yellow, creamy matter....Nat Phos
>> without....Ferr Phos
> thick yellow matter is discharged....Silica
> pus is discharged, when....Calc Sulph

injury
> after....Calc Sulph

pain of....Ferr Phos
iritis-inflammation of iris....Ferr Phos, Kali Mur, Nat Mur, Silica
itching....Kali Sulph, Mag Phos
lachrymal apparatus
    diseases of....Silica
    tear duct obstruction....Nat Mur
lacrimation-secretion and discharge of tears
    acrid....Nat Mur
    burning....Nat Phos, Nat Sulph
    colds in head, associated with....Nat Mur
    eruption of small vesicles, with....Nat Mur
    general, in....Mag Phos, Nat Sulph, Nat Mur
    neuralgic pains, with....Nat Mur, Mag Phos
    open air, on going in....Nat Mur
    profuse....Nat Mur
    weakness, associated with....Nat Mur
    wearing glasses all day, from; creates a sensation of blow-
        ing on the eyes....Calc Fluor
    wind, from, or going into cold air; weak eyes....Nat Mur
lens, dimness of....Kali Sulph
lids (see Eyelids)
light, sensitive to (also see Photophobia)....Mag Phos
Meibomian gland, enlarged....Calc Fluor
mucus discharge (see Eyes, discharge)
muscular, neuralgic pains around eye, with much watering....Nat
    Mur
nervous causes, ailments from....Kali Phos, Mag Phos, Nat Phos
neuralgia
    around eyes; right side worse; may need to add Nat
        Mur....Mag Phos
    ciliary....Nat Mur
    flow of tears, with; can recur daily at certain times....Nat
        Mur
    general, in....Mag Phos, Nat Mur, Calc Phos
    lacrimation, with....Nat Mur
    periodical....Nat Mur
    right side worse....Mag Phos
    right eye, over....Silica
    supraorbital....Mag Phos, Ferr Phos
    warmth relieves....Mag Phos
nystagmus....Mag Phos

orbits, pressure and soreness in....Silica
pain
        acute....Ferr Phos
        aggravated by movement....Ferr Phos
        burning sensation....Ferr Phos, Kali Phos
        excoriation in eyes, sensation of....Nat Mur
        eye, in....Ferr Phos
        eyeball, in; moving aggravates....Ferr Phos
        neuralgic (see Eyes, neuralgia)
        over eye....Nat Phos, Mag Phos, Nat Mur
        smarting; may be tears....Nat Mur
        splinter, feels like....Calc Sulph
        sticks in eye, sensation of....Kali Phos
perceptive power lost after suffering exhaustion....Kali Phos
photophobia (see Photophobia)
ptosis....Kali Phos, Mag Phos
puberty, troubles at....Calc Phos
pupils
        contracted....Mag Phos
        dilated during disease....Kali Phos
pus in anterior chamber; may be smoky....Calc Sulph, Kali Mur,
   Silica
redness
        burning sensation, with....Ferr Phos
        general, in....Ferr Phos, Nat Mur
        inflammation of whites of eyes; eyeballs seem too
          large....Nat Mur
retinitis....Calc Sulph, Kali Mur, Ferr Phos
sand in, feeling of....Kali Mur, Ferr Phos, Kali Phos
sclera/conjunctiva
        dirty yellow color....Nat Phos
        tinged with yellowish color...Nat Sulph
scrofulous inflammation with spots on cornea....Calc Phos
sore....Kali Phos
sparks or flickering lights before eyes....Calc Fluor, Mag Phos,
   Nat Phos
spasms of....Calc Phos, Mag Phos
spots, colors before eyes, or abnormal vision (see Vision)
squinting
        intestinal irritation, from....Nat Phos
        spasmodic....Mag Phos

strabismus, from....Kali Phos, Nat Phos, Mag Phos
staring appearance....Kali Phos
stiff feeling and weakness of the eyes....Calc Phos
strabismus....Kali Phos, Nat Phos, Mag Phos
strain on eyes....Kali Phos, Calc Fluor
styes, kernels, induration of the lids; if chronic condition give
    12X; alternate with Calc Fluor and Ferr Phos for inflammation
    (also see Styes)....Silica
surface, itching on....Calc Fluor
tears (see Eyes, lacrimation)
twitching of....Kali Phos, Mag Phos, Calc Phos
vesicles, eruption of....Nat Mur
vision (see Vision)
watering (see Eyes, lacrimation)

## FACE

ache
    aggravates symptoms
        body gets cold....Mag Phos
        cold wind....Mag Phos
        touch....Mag Phos
        washing....Mag Phos
    ameliorates symptoms (makes symptoms better)
        cold applications....Ferr Phos, Kali Phos
        cool, open air....Kali Sulph
        heat....Mag Phos, Silica
    bed, after going to....Mag Phos
    cheekbone, in....Nat Sulph
    coldness of nape, with....Ferr Phos
    constipation, with....Nat Mur
    cutting pains, with....Mag Phos
    evening, in....Kali Sulph
    exhaustion, great, with....Kali Phos
    flushing, with....Ferr Phos
    general, in....Calc Sulph, Kali Mur, Kali Sulph, Silica,
        Mag Phos, Kali Phos, Ferr Phos
    heated room, in....Kali Sulph
    jaw, lower, right side of....Nat Phos
    lumps or nodules on face, with....Silica
    moving, on....Ferr Phos
    neuralgic....Nat Phos, Kali Phos, Kali Mur

right side, on....Mag Phos, Nat Phos
superior maxillary bone, in....Calc Phos
swelling, from....Kali Mur
tears flowing, with....Nat Mur
aggravations of symptoms at night....Calc Phos
ameliorated by cold compress to the area.....Ferr Phos
anemic person, in....Ferr Phos, Calc Phos
bloated, without fever....Nat Phos
burning sensation....Kali Phos
cheeks
    ache....Nat Sulph
    hot and sore....Ferr Phos
    painful
        aggravated after going to bed....Mag Phos
        general, in....Kali Mur
    sore....Ferr Phos
    suppuration threatens....Calc Sulph
    swelling
        general....Kali Mur, Calc Sulph
        hard....Calc Fluor
chlorotic face....Ferr Phos, Calc Phos
cold
    clammy skin, and....Calc Phos
    numbness of face, and....Calc Phos
    prominent parts, of....Calc Phos
complexion (see Complexion)
contortions from loss of power of facial muscles....Kali Phos
cracked skin....Silica
eruptions (see also Eruptions, Pimples)
    any cause, with discharge....Silica
    chin, on....Nat Mur
    cold sores....Calc Fluor, Nat Mur
    forehead, pustular....Nat Mur
    full of pimples....Calc Sulph, Calc Phos
    herpetic (see Herpes)
    pimples (see Pimples)
    pustules (see Pustules)
    vesicles, covered with (see Vesicles)
epithelioma....Kali Sulph
eyes, sunken, hollow....Kali Phos
features distorted

general, in....Kali Sulph, Kali Phos
red face, with....Kali Sulph
feverish complexion....Ferr Phos
flushed face
    cold sensation at nape of neck, with....Ferr Phos
    easily....Ferr Phos
    fever, with; quick full pulse....Ferr Phos
flushing heat, with....Ferr Phos
freckles....Calc Phos
glands, swollen about jaw and neck....Kali Mur
greasy....Nat Mur, Calc Phos
induration of cellular tissues....Silica
itches....Kali Phos, Nat Mur
jaundice....Nat Sulph
jawbone
    caries of....Silica
    necrosis....Silica
    swelling, hard....Calc Fluor
livid....Kali Phos
lupus....Calc Phos, Silica
muscles, convulsive, twitching....Mag Phos
neuralgia
    aggravates
        cold....Mag Phos
        heated room, being in....Kali Sulph
    evening, worse....Kali Sulph
    exhaustion of nervous system, with....Kali Phos
    flow of tears, with....Nat Mur
    inflammatory....Ferr Phos
    pressing pain....Ferr Phos
    primary remedy....Mag Phos
    prosopalgia....Nat Phos, Mag Phos, Ferr Phos
    relieved
        being in cold air....Kali Sulph
        hot applications, by....Mag Phos
        cold application, with....Ferr Phos
    shifting pain, with....Kali Sulph, Mag Phos
    shooting pains, with....Mag Phos
    spasmodic pains....Mag Phos
    superior maxillary bone, in....Kali Phos, Calc Phos
    tearing, with....Calc Phos, Mag Phos

tears and excessive saliva, with....Kali Phos
throbbing pain....Ferr Phos
worse touch, pressure, cold; right sided....Mag Phos
nodules on face....Calc Sulph
pain
    aggravated after going to bed....Mag Phos
    ameliorates
        cold....Kali Phos
        warmth....Mag Phos
    cheeks, in....Kali Mur
    creeping....Calc Phos
    cutting....Mag Phos
    grinding....Mag Phos, Calc Phos
    heat in face, and....Ferr Phos
    jerking pains in face....Mag Phos
    lightning-like....Mag Phos
    neuralgic (see Face, neuralgia)
pale, sickly, sallow (see also Complexion)....Kali Phos, Calc Phos
paralysis....Kali Phos
red
    fever, without....Nat Phos
    hot, and....Ferr Phos
rheumatism in face....Calc Phos
swelling
    cheeks....Kali Mur
    general, in....Kali Mur
    hard....Calc Fluor
    jawbone....Calc Fluor
    painful....Kali Mur
    parotid gland....Calc Phos
    submaxillary gland....Calc Phos
sweats
    cold, on face....Calc Phos
    while eating....Nat Mur, Kali Phos
tearing....Calc Phos, Mag Phos
tic douloureux....Ferr Phos, Nat Phos, Mag Phos
white about nose and mouth....Nat Mur, Nat Phos

## FAINTNESS

fright or fatigue, from....Kali Phos
general, in....Kali Phos

grief, from....Kali Phos
nervous, sensitive people....Kali Phos
tendency to....Kali Phos

**FASTING**
symptoms
better from fasting....Kali Phos
resulting from fasting....Nat Phos

**FAT ASSIMILATION,** helps with....Nat Phos

**FATIGUE (see also Vitality, Debility)**
abnormally so....Nat Mur
brain (see Brain, fatigue)
easily....Kali Phos, Nat Mur, Ferr Phos
exertion, physical, tires you easily....Ferr Phos
exhaustion
colic, with....Nat Sulph
extreme....Silica, Mag Phos, Kali Phos
irritable, excited, and....Silica
nervous....Kali Phos, Mag Phos
general, in....Calc Phos, Kali Phos, Ferr Phos
listlessness....Silica
mental (see Mental States)
tired in morning....Nat Mur

**FEET (see also Extremities)**
asleep, fall....Nat Mur
burning
general, in....Kali Phos
night, at....Silica, Nat Phos
chapped and fissures where there is a thickened derma;
persistent....Calc Fluor
clammy feeling in, with inability to sleep late in the morning; in
hands also....Calc Phos
cold
chest troubles, with....Calc Phos
day, during; warm at night....Nat Phos
hands, and....Nat Mur, Calc Phos, Kali Sulph
icy, and....Calc Phos, Nat Phos
cracks between toes....Nat Mur
cramping in; if Mag Phos does not relieve give Kali Sulph....Mag Phos
edema....Nat Mur, Nat Sulph, Calc Sulph

fidgety feeling in....Kali Phos
fistulous ulcers about the feet....Calc Phos
itch (see Itching)
pain through feet....Silica
perspiration, chronic, fetid; suppressed perspiration....Silica
soles

>    burning....Calc Sulph, Nat Sulph, Kali Phos, Nat Mur
>    drawing in....Nat Phos, Kali Phos
>    itching....Calc Sulph, Kali Phos
>    pain in....Nat Phos, Kali Phos

sore, hot, aching....Kali Phos, Mag Phos, Silica
spasms; tonic....Silica
sweat, offensive....Silica
sweaty; give at bedtime....Silica
swell....Kali Mur
tender, very....Mag Phos, Silica
tired....Silica
toes

>    cracked and chapped between toes....Nat Mur
>    itching of....Nat Sulph
>    spasm of....Silica

toenails grow inward....Kali Mur, Silica

## FEMALE DISORDERS (see also Sexual Organs, Female)

after confinement when pelvic muscles are relaxed....Calc Fluor
dragging

>    groin, in....Calc Fluor
>    small of back, in....Calc Fluor

general, in....Calc Phos, Ferr Phos
nausea and vomiting after eating; hammering in forehead and
    temples, sleep disturbed with dreams; excessive menstrual
    flow....Ferr Phos

## FEVER

acid symptoms, with....Nat Phos
bilious....Mag Phos, Nat Phos, Nat Sulph
blood poisoning, from....Kali Sulph
brain....Kali Phos
broken bones, when; convalescing and rebuilding health....Ferr
    Phos, Kali Mur
catarrh

>    chilly sensations, with....Ferr Phos

chills and cramps, with....Ferr Phos, Mag Phos
congestion, with....Ferr Phos, Kali Mur
general, in....Ferr Phos, Kali Mur, Nat Sulph
perspiration, to promote....Kali Sulph
quickened pulse, with....Ferr Phos
chills, with
    back, in....Nat Mur
    nervous, with teeth chattering....Mag Phos, Kali Phos
    children, in (see also Children, feverish)
    run up and down spine....Mag Phos
chilliness, with
    begins in morning around 10:00 a.m. and continues
        until noon; preceded by intense heat, thirst, sweat,
        great languor, emaciation, sallow complexion,
        blisters on lips, headache....Nat Mur
    feeling of chilliness, especially in the back; saliva watery;
        full heavy headache; increased heat....Nat Mur
    great, with white coated tongue, constipation....Kali Mur
enteric....Kali Sulph, Kali Mur, Nat Mur, Ferr Phos, Kali Phos
eruptive diseases, with; aids desquamation....Kali Sulph
flushes of heat from digestive causes....Nat Phos
gastric
    first stage....Ferr Phos
    general, in....Kali Phos, Ferr Phos, Kali Sulph, Kali Mur
    temperature rises in evening....Kali Sulph
headache, frontal, from flushes of heat....Nat Phos
heat ameliorates temperature....Silica
high temperature....Ferr Phos
infants; give 1 tablet every hour until fever is gone....Ferr Phos
infections, with....Calc Sulph, Silica
inflammation, with
    first stage....Ferr Phos
    second stage....Kali Mur
initial classic symptoms of flushed face, elevated temperature,
    congestion, hot dry skin....Ferr Phos
intermittent
    acid vomiting, with....Nat Phos
    chronic....Calc Phos
    cramps, with....Mag Phos
    general, in; all stages; vomiting of bile may be
        present....Nat Sulph, Mag Phos, Kali Mur, Nat Mur

perspiration, debilitating....Kali Phos
temperature, high....Ferr Phos
tongue yellow and slimy-coated....Kali Sulph
vomiting of food, with....Ferr Phos
moisture regulating process disturbed, associated with....Nat Mur
nervous....Kali Phos
night sweats, profuse, with....Nat Mur, Calc Phos, Silica, Nat
   Sulph, Ferr Phos, Calc Sulph
perspiration (see also Perspiration)
   clammy on body....Calc Phos
   cold on face....Calc Phos
   day time, excessive....Nat Mur
   excessive, exhausting, while eating; with stomach
      weakness....Kali Phos, Calc Phos
   promotes perspiration to control temperature....Ferr
      Phos, Kali Sulph
   sour smelling....Nat Phos
primary remedies....Ferr Phos, Kali Mur
puerperal....Kali Mur
pulse, quick
   irregular and a high temperature; associated with a gen-
      eral nervous excitement....Kali Phos
   nervous fevers, irregular, with nervous excitement and
      much weakness....Kali Phos
   temperature high....Ferr Phos
recede, when begins to; remedy is a building agent....Kali Mur
remittent....Nat Sulph
rheumatic....Ferr Phos, Nat Mur, Kali Mur
rising temperature in evening....Kali Sulph, Kali Phos, Ferr Phos
saliva clear, watery....Nat Mur
scarlet fever....Kali Phos, Kali Sulph, Kali Mur, Nat Mur, Ferr
   Phos
secondary stage after Ferr Phos....Kali Phos
shivering at beginning of fever....Calc Phos, Ferr Phos
skin dry and hot....Kali Sulph
sleeplessness, with....Kali Phos
stupor, with....Nat Mur, Kali Phos
suppurative process, during....Silica
temperature, high....Ferr Phos
third stage of chronic, catarrhal fevers and inflammation; fevers
   increase during evening and night and remit in the

morning....Kali Sulph

thirst increased....Nat Mur

typhoid fever....Kali Sulph, Kali Mur, Kali Phos, Nat Mur, Ferr Phos

vomiting of sour fluids, during....Nat Phos

yellow fever....Kali Phos, Ferr Phos, Nat Sulph

## FIBROSITIS

acid condition exists; give along with the main indicated
remedy....Nat Phos

acute cases, helpful in....Kali Mur

acute, inflammatory pains caused by suddenly getting chills;
excessive exercise can be stressful to the system....Ferr Phos

general, in....Ferr Phos, Nat Phos, Silica

shifting, fleeting pains....Kali Sulph

toxic fluids, helps eliminate....Nat Sulph

## FINGERNAILS (see Nails)

## FINGERS (see also Hands)

clenched or in a fist....Mag Phos

dislocates easily, phalanges....Calc Fluor

exostosis....Calc Fluor

joints

blisters itching, with....Nat Mur

enlarged....Calc Fluor

inflamed....Ferr Phos, Nat Phos

stiff....Calc Sulph, Nat Sulph

## FIRST-AID

collapse; take 6 of each in a small amount of hot water and sip
frequently....Kali Phos, Mag Phos, Nat Mur

discharge is thick, yellow (see also Discharge)....Silica

hemorrhages....Ferr Phos

injured area, apply to, in powder form....Ferr Phos

shock, for....Nat Sulph, Nat Mur, Kali Phos

swelling, for....Ferr Phos, Kali Mur

wounds that are suppurating....Calc Sulph

## FISSURES

dermal; cracks; persistent....Calc Fluor

general, in....Nat Mur

hands and feet, of, where there is a thickened derma;
persistent....Calc Fluor

tendency to form....Silica, Calc Fluor

FISTULA....Calc Phos, Calc Fluor, Silica

FLATULENCE

    accumulation of gas....Calc Phos

    belching, with; associated with indigestion (see also
        Eructations)....Mag Phos

    colic

        general, in....Nat Phos, Nat Sulph

        green sour-smelling stools, or vomiting of curdled
            masses....Nat Phos

    confinement, after....Nat Sulph

    constitutional remedy; give night and morning....Calc Phos

    digestive problems, with (see also Digestion, Dyspepsia)....Mag
        Phos, Calc Phos, Kali Mur

    distention and constipation, with....Mag Phos

    excessive accumulation of gas in stomach....Calc Phos

    full sensation in stomach....Mag Phos

    heart, disturbance about....Kali Phos, Nat Phos

    heartburn, with (see also Heartburn)....Calc Phos

    indigestion of starchy and fatty foods, due to....Nat Sulph

    liver sluggish....Nat Sulph, Nat Mur, Kali Mur

    meals, after; repeat every 1/2 hour until better....Mag Phos

    menses, during....Nat Sulph

    noisy, offensive....Kali Phos, Calc Phos

    pain, with

        left sided....Kali Phos

        no relief from belching....Mag Phos

        risings sour....Kali Phos, Nat Phos, Nat Sulph, Calc Phos

        stomach distention, with....Mag Phos

        sulfurous odor....Kali Sulph

        taste of food comes back....Ferr Phos

        troublesome....Mag Phos

FLUIDS

    excess water, eliminates....Nat Sulph

    poison-charged fluids, removes....Nat Sulph

    protects against; believed to coat surfaces such as the stomach
        wall, eyeballs, nasal passages, mouth, throat, bladder and other
        organs needing protection against moisture....Calc Sulph

FLUSH, easily....Ferr Phos

FOLLICULAR INFILTRATIONS....Kali Mur

FONTANELLES, lack closure in infants....Calc Phos

FRACTURES OF BONES

    healing, to promote....Calc Phos, Ferr Phos

    mending, increases; give in all cases when there is injury or
        brittleness of the bones....Calc Phos

    non-union....Ferr Phos

FROSTBITE

    circulation poor, due to....Calc Phos

    compress, apply locally; renew as needed; take also internally....Calc
        Phos, Calc Fluor, Kali Mur, Kali Phos, Nat Sulph

    exudate is thin, yellow....Kali Sulph

    general, in....Kali Mur, Kali Phos

    hands and feet, on....Kali Mur, Kali Phos

    irritation, helps with—Kali Phos

    itch and tingle, that....Kali Phos

    nutritional deficiency, due to....Calc Phos

    pain and inflammation, with....Kali Mur, Ferr Phos

    skin, cracks in....Calc Fluor

    swelling, with....Kali Mur

    tingling and irritation, with....Kali Phos

FUNGUS

    bleeds easily....Silica

    general, in....Kali Sulph

    malignant, bleeding growth....Nat Mur

    rashes....Kali Sulph

    tinea capitis; tinea in general....Kali Sulph

GAIT, unsteady....Nat Phos

GALL BLADDER TROUBLE....Nat Sulph

GALL STONES

    colic; better results when given in hot water; take as
        needed....Mag Phos

    general, in....Nat Phos, Nat Sulph, Silica

    prevents formation....Calc Phos

    spasms from....Mag Phos

GANGLION

    general, in....Calc Fluor, Calc Phos

    wrist, at back of....Calc Fluor

**GANGRENE,** if suppuration is desired give Silica; salts may be dissolved in water and used as a compress; don't apply hot....Kali Phos, Calc Sulph, Kali Mur, Nat Phos

**GAS** (see Flatulence)

**GASTRALGIA** (see Stomach, Ache)

**GASTRIC DISTURBANCES** (see also Dyspepsia, Digestion)
    abrasions....Nat Phos
    fatty food, due to....Kali Mur
    fever, with....Ferr Phos
    general, in....Kali Sulph
    liver symptoms, associated with; jaundice skin; pain in right side; flatulence, diarrhea....Nat Sulph
    pains....Kali Mur
    regurgitation after eating....Mag Phos
    sensation of band around body....Mag Phos
    tight clothing about waist, unbearable....Nat Sulph, Ferr Phos
    ulcerations....Kali Phos, Nat Phos
    weakness; giving rise to acidity....Calc Phos

**GASTRIC ULCER**....Nat Phos, Kali Phos, Kali Mur

**GASTRITIS**
    chronic....Kali Sulph
    drinking hot liquids, from....Kali Mur
    gastrointestinal disturbances, associated with....Ferr Phos, Kali Mur
    general, in; if increased acidity replace Kali Sulph with Nat Phos....Ferr Phos, Kali Mur, Kali Phos, Kali Sulph
    jaundice, after....Kali Sulph

**GASTROINTESTINAL DISTURBANCES**
    acidity symptoms, with....Nat Phos
    aggravated by tight clothing....Nat Sulph, Ferr Phos
    assimilation and digestion, helps; take other remedies....Calc Phos
    disposition, irritable and fretful....Nat Phos
    dyspepsia, with hot, flushed face (see also Dyspepsia)....Ferr Phos
    fatty or rich foods, associated with eating....Kali Mur
    gastritis, associated with....Ferr Phos, Kali Mur
    heartburn after eating (see also Heartburn)....Nat Phos
    pain, swelling and tenderness of the stomach, with....Ferr Phos
    sensation of band around body....Mag Phos

tongue (see Tongue, coating)

vomiting of undigested food; tongue is clean....Ferr Phos

## GENITAL WEAKNESS AND SEXUAL NEURASTHENIA

(see Sexual Organs)

## GIDDINESS

gastric derangements, from....Nat Phos

working for long periods of time in a kneeling position and them standing up....Ferr Phos

## GINGIVITIS (see Gums)

## GLANDS

congestion of....Kali Mur

enlarged

> lymphoid structures: tonsils, adenoids, cervical, axillary, inguinal and other glands....Calc Fluor
>
> suppurating....Silica

external, painful....Calc Phos

hardened anywhere....Calc Fluor

indurated....Calc Fluor

inflamed....Ferr Phos

painful, aching....Calc Phos

scrofulous infiltration of....Kali Mur

suppurating....Silica, Calc Sulph

swellings and enlargements

> acute; primary remedy....Kali Mur
>
> cervical....Nat Phos, Kali Mur
>
> chronic....Calc Phos
>
> inguinal....Silica
>
> mesenteric....Calc Phos
>
> soft; primary remedy....Kali Mur
>
> submaxillary....Nat Mur
>
> suppuration
>
>> general, in....Calc Sulph, Silica
>>
>> salivary gland, of....Silica
>>
>> sebaceous glands, of....Silica
>
> thyroid....Nat Mur, Calc Fluor, Silica, Calc Phos
>
> tongue, under....Nat Mur
>
> ulceration of....Ferr Phos, Calc Sulph

GLAUCOMA (see Eyes)

GLOSSITIS (see Tongue, Inflammation)

GOITER

general, in....Calc Fluor, Nat Phos, Calc Phos, Nat Mur, Silica
watery secretions, with.....Nat Mur

GONORRHEA

anemia, with....Calc Phos
chronic....Silica, Nat Mur, Nat Sulph, Kali Phos, Calc Phos
discharge

bloody....Ferr Phos, Kali Phos
creamy, golden-yellow....Nat Phos
greenish....Kali Sulph, Nat Sulph
purulent....Calc Sulph
slimy....Nat Mur, Kali Sulph
transparent....Nat Mur
yellow....Kali Sulph
watery....Nat Mur

exudation

intestinal....Kali Mur
subcutaneous....Kali Mur

first remedy given....Nat Phos
inflammatory stage....Ferr Phos
itching, with....Calc Phos
orchitis from suppressed gonorrhea....Kali Mur, Kali Sulph
ovarian inflammation from gonorrhea....Nat Phos, Kali Mur
suppressed....Nat Sulph
swelling, for....Kali Mur

GOUT

acute attacks....Ferr Phos, Nat Sulph, Nat Phos, Nat Mur
chronic; may have profuse, sour smelling sweat....Nat Mur, Nat
Sulph, Nat Phos
dissolves the urate of soda found in deposits and is flushed
through the lymphatic system....Silica
enlargement, gouty, of the finger joints....Calc Fluor
excess of uric acid....Silica, Kali Mur
feet, when in; acute and chronic....Nat Sulph
inflammatory stages, during....Ferr Phos
joints, in....Calc Phos
onset of condition....Ferr Phos

pain
>general, in....Kali Mur, Mag Phos, Nat Mur, Calc Phos
>motion brings on....Kali Mur
>severe....Mag Phos, Kali Mur
periodical attacks of....Nat Mur
primary remedy....Nat Sulph
profuse or sour sweating, with....Nat Phos
rheumatic; aggravated at night....Calc Phos
stomach involvement, if....Nat Phos
swelling
>general, in....Kali Mur
>uric acid deposits, due to....Nat Phos
urates lodging around joints and muscles, breaks up....Silica
uric acid deposits; stiffness, swelling, and other rheumatic symptoms....Nat Phos

GRANULATIONS, excessive....Calc Sulph

GRAVEL, primary remedy; include Nat Phos with excessive acidity....Nat Sulph

GROIN PAIN (see Sexual Organs)

GROWTHS
cancerous....Kali Sulph
osseous....Calc Fluor

GROWING PAINS in children....Ferr Phos

GROWTH, aids; helps with normal development....Calc Phos

GUMBOILS
before
>matter forms....Kali Mur, Nat Mur
>pus begins to form....Kali Mur
general, in....Silica, Calc Fluor, Kali Mur, Nat Mur
hard swelling on jaw, with; dissolve salts in mouth slowly....Calc Fluor
suppuration....Calc Sulph, Silica

GUMS
bleed
>easily....Nat Mur, Kali Phos, Calc Sulph
>general, in....Kali Phos, Nat Mur
>predisposition to....Kali Phos

routine brushing, during....Calc Sulph, Silica

tendency to....Kali Phos, Nat Mur

blisters on....Nat Sulph

boils, with hard jaw swellings....Calc Fluor

burning....Nat Sulph

gingivitis; caused by deposits of bile in the mouth    Nat Sulph

inflamed; hot and swollen....Ferr Phos, Calc Phos

painful

general, in....Calc Phos, Kali Sulph, Kali Mur

slight pressure on gums, with; abscess at the
roots....Silica

pale....Calc Phos, Kali Sulph

pyorrhea (see Pyorrhea)

red, bright seam on....Kali Phos

sensitive

cold water, to....Mag Phos

general, in....Nat Mur, Silica

pressure or touch, to....Ferr Phos, Mag Phos

sore....Calc Fluor, Kali Mur

spongy, receding....Kali Phos

suppuration, to promote....Calc Fluor, Silica

swollen

burning and red....Kali Phos

inside, on the, and with soreness....Calc Sulph

ulcerated....Nat Mur

white....Kali Sulph

## HAIR

conditioner; for impoverished conditions of the hair and lack of
luster....Silica

falling out (see Alopecia)

healthy, retaining....Silica

pain on combing hair....Ferr Phos, Nat Sulph

primary remedy for hair problems....Silica

sycosis-chronic inflammation of hair follicles....Nat Sulph, Silica,
Nat Mur

## HAMSTRINGS (see also Muscles)

painful contractions of....Nat Mur

sore....Nat Phos

## HANDS (see also Extremities)

burning and itching....Kali Sulph

chapped from the cold....Ferr Phos, Calc Fluor

chapped, fissures; where there is a thickened derma;
    persistent....Calc Fluor

clammy feeling, with inability to sleep late in the morning; may
    be found in the feet....Calc Phos

cold

>   general, in....Nat Mur
>
>   feet, and....Nat Mur, Calc Phos, Kali Sulph

cramping

>   general, in; give Kali Sulph if Mag Phos doesn't
>       relieve....Mag Phos
>
>   writing, while....Calc Phos, Mag Phos, Nat Phos

fingers (see Fingers)

itch (see Itching)

palms

>   chapped, cracks; apply remedies also topically....Calc
>       Fluor, Calc Sulph
>
>   fissured; apply remedies topically....Calc Fluor, Calc Sulph
>
>   hot....Ferr Phos
>
>   itch....Kali Phos
>
>   raw and sore....Nat Sulph
>
>   warts in....Kali Mur, Nat Mur, Nat Sulph

shaking involuntary....Mag Phos

skin is burning and itching....Kali Sulph

spasms; tonic....Silica

thumbs drawn in....Mag Phos

trembling

>   involuntary....Mag Phos
>
>   writing, while....Nat Sulph, Mag Phos

HANDWRITING, unsteady....Mag Phos

HANGNAILS....Nat Mur, Silica

HARDNESS, stony; anywhere in the body....Calc Fluor

HAWKING (see Cough), constant

HAY FEVER

congestion, with; inflammation and headache present....Ferr Phos

craving for salt, associated with; worse exposure to sun....Nat Mur

depression, with; helps breathing....Kali Phos

dryness with a tickling cough; worse cold drinks, lying down at
    night, speaking....Silica

general, in; sniffing a watered-down solution several times a day
may also be helpful....Nat Mur, Nat Sulph, Ferr Phos, Kali
Phos, Mag Phos, Silica

itching and tingling in nose

 violent sneezing, with, and excoriating discharge;
 hoarseness; roughness; onset on damp, chilly day or a
 hot, humid day....Nat Sulph, Silica

 watery discharge, with....Nat Mur

pollen from hay fields, especially....Nat Mur

prevents threatening attacks or helps to relax during attack; worse
if weather has been sultry and stuffy during the day; if
oppressed with short anxious breathing, give remedy every
hour during the day and throughout the evening in hot
water....Mag Phos

spasms relax, helps....Mag Phos

sun exposure, after....Nat Mur

## HEAD

bones, large, separated....Calc Phos

bruising pain in....Ferr Phos

burning sensation in top of....Nat Sulph

cerebral apoplexy....Silica

colds (see Colds)

cold to touch, feels....Calc Phos

crawling feeling over the head, with cold sensation....Calc Phos

falls or injuries, effects of....Nat Sulph

fontanelles remain open....Silica, Calc Phos

fullness of....Calc Phos

heat in vertex....Nat Sulph, Nat Phos

heaviness of head in morning after waking; giddiness and
dullness....Nat Mur

hydrocephalus....Calc Phos, Kali Phos, Nat Mur

inability to hold up head....Calc Phos

injury due to falling, worse since; may need high homeopathic
doses; helps with mental troubles associated with falls on and
injuries to the head....Nat Sulph

involuntary shaking of....Mag Phos, Kali Phos

lumps on....Calc Fluor

nods forward involuntarily....Nat Mur

nodules on....Silica

noises in (see Ears, noises)

old head injuries....Nat Sulph
pain (see Headache)
pressure, intense, with heat and nausea....Nat Phos
pressure upon....Calc Phos
rush of blood to head....Ferr Phos
scalp (see Scalp)
sensation
    head would open, as if....Nat Mur
    pressure, of....Nat Sulph
    weight at back of head, as if....Kali Phos
sensitive to cold air....Ferr Phos
skull, thin and soft....Calc Phos
sore
    back of head....Kali Phos
    touch, to....Ferr Phos
spasms....Mag Phos
sweat, in children....Silica, Calc Phos
swellings, hard....Calc Fluor
tearing sensation in bones of skull....Calc Phos
trembling of; involuntary shaking....Kali Phos, Mag Phos
ulcers on top of head (see also Ulcerations)....Calc Phos

## HEADACHE

abdominal irritation, from....Silica
aggravates symptoms
    change in weather....Calc Phos
    cold....Calc Phos, Mag Phos
    evening....Kali Sulph
    exertion....Silica
    heat....Calc Phos
    heated room....Kali Sulph
    light....Silica
    loss of sleep....Kali Phos
    mental exertion....Silica, Mag Phos, Calc Phos, Kali Phos
    mornings....Nat Mur
    motion....Ferr Phos, Nat Sulph
    moving head from side to side or backward....Kali Sulph
    noise....Silica, Ferr Phos
    pressure as from a hat....Calc Phos
    reading....Nat Sulph
    shaking head....Ferr Phos

stooping....Ferr Phos
stuffy atmosphere....Kali Sulph
studying....Silica
warm atmosphere; evening; aches in back, neck,
    limbs....Kali Sulph
warm room....Kali Sulph
ameliorates symptoms (makes symptoms better)
    cheerful excitement....Kali Phos
    cold applications....Ferr Phos
    cool, open air....Kali Sulph
    eating....Nat Phos, Kali Phos
    heat....Mag Phos
    motion....Kali Phos
    nosebleed....Ferr Phos
    quiet....Nat Sulph
    warm applications always relieve symptoms....Mag Phos
    warmth; wrapping up head warmly....Silica
around head....Calc Sulph
awakens in morning with headache....Nat Phos
begins in
        evening....Kali Sulph
        morning....Nat Mur, Nat Sulph, Nat Phos
biliousness, with....Nat Sulph
bitter taste in the mouth with nausea; worse with damp, warm
    weather; sick headache....Nat Sulph
brain feels as if it were swishing about....Mag Phos
cachectic persons, of....Silica, Nat Mur
catarrhal....Nat Mur
centered in top of head....Nat Sulph, Ferr Phos
children; chief remedies....Ferr Phos, Calc Phos
chills up and down spine, with....Mag Phos
chronic
        general, in....Silica, Nat Mur, Calc Phos
        nausea and vomiting that usually begins in the morning,
            settles in the forehead by noon; feels head will burst;
            worse mental exertion, light, noise, cold air and
            moving head....Silica
        occasional; especially worse in morning; better in open
            air....Calc Sulph
cold feeling in head, with....Calc Phos, Silica
cold, from....Ferr Phos

confusion, with....Kali Phos
congestive....Ferr Phos, Silica, Nat Sulph, Nat Mur
constipation, with....Nat Mur, Kali Mur
crown of the head, on; awakening; sick headache with acid
   symptoms; follows wine or milk consumption....Nat Phos, Nat
   Sulph, Mag Phos, Nat Mur
dentition, during (see also Teething)....Calc Phos
despondency, with....Kali Phos
diarrhea, bilious, with....Nat Sulph
dizziness, with....Nat Sulph
drowsiness....Nat Mur
dull
     general, in....Nat Mur, Calc Phos
     heavy, and....Ferr Phos, Nat Mur
     right-sided....Ferr Phos
     top of head, on....Ferr Phos
dizziness; worse warm room; worse evening....Kali Sulph
dull, heavy, with drowsiness; not refreshed on waking....Nat Mur
empty feeling in stomach, with....Kali Phos
exam time; especially helpful for students who develop headaches
   at exam time....Kali Phos
exhaustion, from....Kali Phos
eyes, over; all phosphate cell salts are recommended....Kali Phos,
   Ferr Phos
flatulence, with....Calc Phos
fluids, loss of, from....Calc Phos, Nat Mur
forehead
     flushes of heat, from....Nat Phos
     noon until evening....Silica
     skull feels a sensation of fullness; accompanied by
       indigestion....Nat Phos, Nat Sulph
     temples, dull, heavy; may include a bursting pain in the
       forehead; worse morning, mental exertion, sitting or
       lying down....Nat Mur
     worse in....Calc Sulph
forgetfulness, with....Calc Phos
frontal (see Headache, forehead)
full, too, feeling as if skull was....Nat Phos
gastric....Silica, Nat Sulph, Calc Phos
gastrointestinal disturbances and sluggish liver, with....Kali Mur
general, in; better results may result if salts are dissolved in hot

water and sipped frequently; check out contributing
causes....Kali Phos, Mag Phos, Nat Phos, Nat Mur, Calc Sulph
gnawing at base of brain....Nat Sulph
gouty predisposition, with....Nat Sulph, Ferr Phos
hawking up,
> white mucus....Kali Mur
> watery mucus....Nat Mur
heavy sensation....Nat Mur
hunger, with....Silica, Kali Phos
inability for thought, with....Kali Phos
indigestion of starchy and fatty foods, flatulence, associated
with....Nat Sulph
injuries to the head, from....Nat Sulph
intermittent....Mag Phos
irritability and fatigue, brought on by or in connection
with....Kali Phos
lasts until noon....Nat Mur
lumps on scalp, accompanied by....Silica
menstruation, associated with (see Menstruation, headache)
mental exertion, resulting from too much....Kali Phos, Silica,
Mag Phos
migraine; general, in; acute attacks; dissolve 6 tablets of each in a
cup of hot water and sip frequently; avoid fats, especially
animal; adopt an acid-free diet; hot foot baths are
helpful....Kali Phos, Mag Phos, Nat Phos, Nat Sulph, Nat
Mur, Silica, Ferr Phos
nape of neck, coming up from....Silica
nape of neck and vertex of head, in....Mag Phos, Silica
nausea, with
> chilliness, and....Mag Phos
> faint from hunger, with....Kali Phos
> faint in afternoon; better evening....Calc Fluor
> general, in....Calc Sulph, Nat Phos
> profuse....Ferr Phos
nervous exhaustion, from....Silica, Kali Phos, Mag Phos
nervous, with sparks before eyes....Mag Phos
nervousness, due to; empty feeling in the pit of the stomach; eating may help; often related to conditions that cause
depression....Kali Phos
neuralgic
> general, in....Mag Phos, Kali Phos

humming in ears, with; better cheerful excitement;
worse being alone; tearful....Kali Phos, Ferr Phos
sharp pain, with....Mag Phos
noise, sensitive to....Kali Phos
occipital....Nat Sulph, Nat Phos, Silica, Mag Phos, Kali Phos
oppressive; better morning, evening; eyes full of tears; sneezing;
dry heat in in nose; some coughing....Ferr Phos
optical defects....Mag Phos
overheating causes....Silica
pains

   beating and bruising sensation....Ferr Phos
   blinding....Ferr Phos
   burning and throbbing....Calc Phos
   colicky....Nat Sulph
   darting; better warmth....Mag Phos
   excruciating....Mag Phos
   hair, in, when combing....Nat Sulph, Ferr Phos
   hammering
      general, in; dull, heavy....Ferr Phos, Nat Mur
      hammers pounding, feels like; worse
         mornings....Nat Mur
   nail driven in, as if....Ferr Phos
   sharp, in nape of neck....Mag Phos
   shifting....Kali Sulph, Mag Phos
   shooting, sharp; better warmth....Mag Phos
   stabbing; better warmth....Mag Phos
   stinging....Mag Phos
   temples, in....Ferr Phos, Nat Phos
   throbbing....Ferr Phos, Silica
   top of head, on....Nat Sulph, Ferr Phos
   vice, as if the head were in; feels as if a metal band has
      been put around the head....Kali Sulph
   violent, at base of brain....Nat Sulph
   weight in back part of head, with weariness and exhaus-
      tion....Kali Phos
periodical....Nat Mur
pressure, intense, with heat and nausea....Nat Phos
prostrated feeling....Kali Phos
puberty age females, of....Calc Phos, Nat Mur
pulsation on top of head....Nat Sulph
red eyes and face, accompanied by....Ferr Phos

rheumatic; worse evening....Kali Sulph

rheumatism accompanies....Calc Phos

right-sided....Ferr Phos

rush of blood to head, from....Ferr Phos

saliva, profuse, in mouth....Nat Mur

school girls, in....Nat Mur, Calc Phos

scrofulous people, in....Silica

sensitive head

>> noise, to....Kali Phos

>> very; throbbing and burning....Calc Phos

scalp soreness, with....Ferr Phos

sick

>> acid symptoms, with, especially following wine or milk consumption....Nat Phos, Nat Sulph, Mag Phos, Nat Mur

>> bilious diarrhea, with....Nat Sulph

>> bitter taste in mouth; vomiting of bile; bilious diarrhea....Nat Sulph

>> constipation, with....Nat Mur

>> gastric problems, from....Nat Sulph

>> general, in....Nat Sulph

>> skull feels too full....Nat Phos

>> sluggish liver, from; tongue coated white; frequent constipation....Kali Mur

>> soreness of scalp; associated with biliousness....Ferr Phos

>> sour vomiting, with....Nat Phos

>> vomiting of undigested food, with....Ferr Phos

sleeplessness, with....Kali Phos, Ferr Phos

sore to touch with bloodshot eyes that are red and inflamed....Ferr Phos

spasmodic symptoms, tendency to....Mag Phos

sparks before eyes, with    Mag Phos

stomach, in....Nat Phos

strength, loss of....Calc Phos, Kali Phos

stretching, when....Kali Phos

students, of....Kali Phos

sun heat, from....Ferr Phos

surrounds entire head....Calc Sulph

sutures, worse near....Calc Phos

tearful mood, with....Kali Phos

tears, profusion of, with....Nat Mur

television, from watching....Calc Phos
ten-eleven a.m.; four-five p.m.....Mag Phos
tightness feeling in head....Mag Phos
tongue (see also Tongue)
    frothy coating on....Nat Mur
    furred....Ferr Phos
    white-coated; gastrointestinal disturbances; sluggish
      liver....Kali Mur
top of head, on; general, in....Ferr Phos, Nat Sulph
top of head, on, with heat....Nat Phos
vertigo
    anemia, with....Calc Phos
    general, in....Ferr Phos, Silica, Nat Sulph
    nausea, and; pain surrounds entire head....Calc Sulph
vomiting
    acid sour fluids....Nat Phos
    bile....Nat Sulph
    food, of....Ferr Phos
    general, in....Kali Mur
    phlegm, transparent....Nat Mur, Calc Phos
    slimy....Nat Phos
    sour matter....Nat Phos
    undigested food....Ferr Phos, Nat Phos
    weariness, with....Kali Phos
    white mucus....Kali Mur
    yawning, with....Kali Phos
walking, while....Nat Mur
weariness, with....Kali Phos
wine consumption, after....Nat Phos
whole head, over....Calc Sulph
worn out, from being....Kali Phos
yawning and stretching, with....Kali Phos

HEARING (see Ears)

HEART

action
    intermittent....Nat Mur, Kali Phos
    weak, causing dizziness....Kali Phos
beat altered....Mag Phos
burn (see Heartburn, Dyspepsia)
cardiac neuroses, associated with tachycardia, palpitation, vertigo

or faintness; spells brought on by mental or physical exertion, or by emotional upset; remedy will not correct the mechanical problem....Kali Phos

carditis....Ferr Phos

constriction about....Nat Mur

degenerating....Kali Phos

dilation....Ferr Phos, Calc Fluor

disease, chronic....Silica

distress about....Kali Phos

endocarditis (see Endocarditis)

excitable easily....Mag Phos

fatty....Kali Phos

fluttering about....Nat Phos, Nat Mur

foramen ovale, non-closure of....Calc Phos

hypertrophy....Nat Mur

muscle weakness; check out contributing causes....Kali Phos, Calc Fluor, Silica

pain

        around heart, during inspiration....Calc Phos

        base of heart, at....Nat Phos

        chest, in (see your Doctor immediately)

            primary remedies; drop 6 tablets of each into a cup of warm water, dissolve, and sip....Mag Phos, Kali Phos

            secondary remedies....Ferr Phos, Kali Mur

        inspiration, during....Calc Phos

        suddenly goes to heart....Nat Phos

palpitations (see Palpitations)

pericarditis....Calc Sulph, Kali Mur, Ferr Phos

pulse (see Pulse)

tone weak....Kali Phos, Mag Phos

trembling about heart....Nat Phos

trouble

        acute pain, with; give every 15 minutes....Calc Fluor

        consoled, not wanting to be; worse with heat; tired and exhausted in morning; likes salty foods and sweets; skin sallow and yellow....Nat Mur

        everything connected with heart problems can be treated with Kali Phos along with whatever else is prescribed....Kali Phos

vital to the action of the heart....Kali Phos

HEARTBURN (see also Dyspepsia)

eating, after; associated with gastrointestinal disturbances (see also Gastrointestinal Disturbances)....Nat Phos

flatulence, with....Calc Phos

gastric fermentation, due to, with slow digestion (see also Digestion)....Nat Mur

gastritis, associated with....Kali Mur, Ferr Phos

mornings; likes salty foods, sweets; skin sallow, yellow....Nat Mur

pain, with....Ferr Phos

HEMORRHAGES

bright red blood....Ferr Phos, Calc Fluor

dark blood....Ferr Phos, Kali Mur

dark clotted blood; vomiting of blood....Kali Mur

first-aid remedy....Ferr Phos

stomach, from....Kali Mur, Ferr Phos

thin and watery....Ferr Phos, Nat Mur

weak, thin, delicate people; blackish blood; looks like coffee grounds....Kali Phos Hemorrhoids

HEMORRHOIDS

aids in healing; apply powdered tablets directly to the bleeding parts....Ferr Phos

anemia, associated with....Calc Fluor, Calc Phos

bleeding....Calc Fluor, Kali Mur, Ferr Phos, Calc Fluor

blind....Kali Sulph, Calc Fluor

chronic....Calc Phos

compress, use as, and swab area; dissolve some tablets in a small amount of water and apply directly with a cotton swab; can be used as a compress to the anus and held all night with suitable bandage....Calc Fluor

constipation, with (see Constipation)

cutting, lightning-like pain....Mag Phos

dark, clotted blood exuded....Kali Mur

external....Kali Sulph

general, in; tablets may be dissolved in warm water and used as a compress when cooled....Calc Fluor, Ferr Phos, Nat Mur, Kali Sulph

inflammation and bleeding, with; apply some powdered tablets directly to the bleeding parts; aids in the healing....Ferr Phos

internal, blind piles; accompanied by pain in the back....Calc
Fluor, Kali Sulph
itching and bleeding; take with other salts indicated....Calc Phos
oozing....Calc Phos
painful, intensely....Kali Phos, Silica
smarting....Nat Mur
stinging....Nat Mur
swollen and hard....Calc Fluor

**HEMOGLOBIN, deficient....Ferr Phos**

**HEPATIC (see Liver)**

**HERNIA....Calc Fluor, Calc Phos, Ferr Phos, Silica**

**HERPES**
acute....Calc Phos, Calc Sulph, Nat Mur
anus, about....Nat Mur
chronic....Calc Phos
circular....Nat Mur
elbow, on....Nat Mur
face, on....Calc Sulph, Nat Mur
general, in; tablets dissolved in water and applied directly to the
lesion with cotton swab....Calc Sulph, Kali Sulph, Nat Mur
knee, bend of....Nat Mur
lips, on; lesion hard....Calc Fluor
nose, around....Silica
palms, in....Kali Sulph
shingles (see Shingles)
vaginal....Calc Sulph
Zoster; take homeopathic Rhus tox 30X at same time....Nat Mur

**HICCUPS**
eating fast, associated with; alternate with Mag Phos if spasms
persist....Nat Mur
general, in; dissolve 10 tablets in hot water and sip
frequently....Mag Phos, Calc Fluor, Nat Mur
stubborn cases; take tablets in a small amount of hot water and
sip....Mag Phos
suffer from....Calc Fluor
vomiting, with....Calc Fluor

**HIP (see also Joints)**
joint disease....Silica, Calc Sulph, Kali Mur, Ferr Phos, Calc Phos,
Nat Mur

pain....Nat Mur, Kali Phos

stitches in left side....Nat Sulph

HIVES

creamy exudate, with....Nat Phos

dry skin and tendency to scale....Kali Sulph

fever, with....Ferr Phos

general, in; can be applied topically....Nat Phos, Kali Phos, Ferr Phos, Nat Sulph, Nat Mur, Mag Phos

pain of....Nat Mur

nettlerash; if in great distress dissolve 6 tablets of each salt in hot water and sip frequently; can also be applied topically....Kali Phos, Mag Phos, Nat Mur, Nat Sulph, Nat Phos

overheated, after being....Nat Mur

rose-colored rash....Nat Phos

soreness of the skin and acidity symptoms, with....Nat Phos

watery, clear eruptions, with....Nat Mur

HOARSENESS

chronic....Calc Sulph

cold, from....Kali Sulph, Ferr Phos, Kali Mur

constant....Calc Phos

coughing, from....Kali Sulph

croupy....Kali Sulph, Kali Mur

dry throat, with; loss of voice (also see Voice)....Ferr Phos

over-exertion of voice, from....Calc Phos

speakers and singers, of....Ferr Phos

HUMIDITY, conditions associated with....Nat Sulph

HUMMING AND BUZZING IN EARS (see Ears, noises)

HUNGER (see Appetite)

HYDROCELE....Calc Fluor

HYDROCEPHALUS (see Head)

HYDROCHLORHYDRIA....Nat Mur, Nat Phos

ILL-NOURISHED STATES....Calc Phos

IMPOTENCE (see Sexual Organs)

INCONTINENCE OF URINE (see Enuresis, Bed Wetting, Bladder Disorders)

INDIGESTION (see Dyspepsia, Gastric Disturbances, Digestion)

INDURATIONS....Calc Fluor

## INFANT'S PROBLEMS

chafed skin....Nat Mur, Nat Phos
constipation (see Constipation)
development, poor....Silica
diarrhea (see Diarrhea)
digestive (see also Digestion)....Nat Phos, Mag Phos
feverish; give 1 tablet every hour until fever is gone if under 2
    years old; over 2 years give 2 tablets (see Fevers)....Ferr Phos
fontanelles, lack of closure....Calc Phos, Silica
foramen ovale, non-closure of....Calc Phos
general; primary remedies....Ferr Phos, Kali Mur, Nat Sulph
growth of tissues, bones and teeth, for....Calc Phos
head affected; add the following remedy to other indicated
    ones....Kali Sulph
influenza; dissolve 10 of each in a cup of hot water; take teaspoon
    doses every hour until fever stops, then reduce
    frequency....Ferr Phos, Kali Mur, Nat Sulph
irritability....Kali Phos, Mag Phos
nursing (see Nursing)
pains in limbs/bones; add other indicated remedies....Kali Mur
vomits
        as soon as infant nurses....Silica, Calc Phos, Ferr Phos
        general, in....Calc Phos
        sour, curdled milk....Calc Phos, Nat Phos
watery symptoms....Nat Mur

## INFECTIONS

fever, with....Calc Sulph, Silica
general, in....Calc Phos
putrid states....Kali Phos
restorative powers after illness....Calc Phos

## INFERTILITY (see Sexual Organs)

## INFILTRATIONS, watery....Nat Sulph

## INFLAMMATION

first stage....Ferr Phos
burning pain....Ferr Phos, Kali Sulph
conditions; to promote perspiration....Kali Sulph

discharge, with (see Discharge, Exudation)
disease; alternate with Ferr Phos, especially with respiratory
    problems such as colds, sore throats, tonsillitis,
    bronchitis....Kali Mur
exudation, beginning of....Kali Mur
fever and heat, for....Ferr Phos
gangrenous....Silica, Kali Phos
general; give first, especially in early stages before exudation
    occurs; Silica is also important....Ferr Phos
hardening after....Calc Fluor
infection, with (see Infection)
pain
        general, in....Ferr Phos
        redness in parts, and....Ferr Phos
        wandering....Kali Sulph
    severe, in chronic ailments....Kali Mur
    skin and internal inflammation....Kali Sulph
    yellow, watery exudation....Nat Sulph
INFLUENZA
    after the flu, give....Nat Sulph
    catarrhal symptoms, with (see also Catarrh); alternate with other
        indicated remedies....Kali Mur
    convalescence, during....Calc Phos, Kali Phos
    discharge (see Discharge)
    fever, with; take every hour until fever subsides....Nat Sulph, Ferr
        Phos, Kali Mur
    general, in; give every 30 minutes....Nat Sulph, Ferr Phos, Kali
        Mur, Nat Mur
    infants, in (see Infant's Problems)
    inflammation and feverish, with....Ferr Phos
    limb pains, with....Kali Mur
    perspiration, promotes; helps control temperature....Kali Sulph
    primary remedy; alternate with Ferr Phos throughout feverish
        stage....Nat Sulph
INGROWN TOENAILS (see Nails)
INJURIES (see also Accidents, First Aid)
    blows, effects of....Kali Mur, Ferr Phos
    head, to, with mental derangement....Nat Sulph
    mechanical....Ferr Phos
    neglected cases of....Calc Sulph

suppurating skin, not yet; apply also externally on injured
   area....Calc Sulph, Ferr Phos
wounds (see Wounds)

## INSECT BITES

effects of; apply externally by moistening a few tablets with water
   and apply externally with cotton; a salve also works well....Nat
   Mur
knees, ankles, and elbow, especially; apply on water soaked cotton
   swabs; may look rash-like....Mag Phos

## INSOMNIA

emotional turmoil, caused by....Mag Phos
excitement, from....Kali Phos, Ferr Phos, Nat Phos
exhaustion, from....Mag Phos
indigestion causes....Nat Phos
nervousness, due to....Kali Phos, Mag Phos
restless sleeping, with....Nat Phos
sleepy during the day, wakeful at night....Calc Sulph
worries about problems, due to....Kali Phos, Ferr Phos

## INTESTINAL

disorders....Kali Sulph
duodenal
         catarrh....Kali Mur
         ulcer....Nat Mur, Nat Sulph, Kali Phos, Ferr Phos
malabsorption....Mag Phos
ulcers....Calc Sulph

## IRRITABILITY

banishes....Kali Phos
biliousness, especially due to....Nat Sulph
easily irritated, especially with yourself....Ferr Phos
exaggerated, all conditions; convulsions, neuralgia, spasmodic,
   coughs, chorea, bladder spasms, sciatica, cardiac
   palpitation....Mag Phos
general, in....Kali Phos, Silica, Mag Phos, Nat Phos, Nat Sulph
trifles, especially people fussing, a clock ticking....Nat Mur

## ITCHING

acid state of blood causes itching of nose and anus....Nat Phos
all over body....Mag Phos, Nat Phos
anus
         general, in; eliminate all citrus juice....Calc Phos, Nat

Phos, Calc Fluor, Kali Sulph, Nat Sulph, Kali Phos
night aggravation....Nat Phos
burning, as from nettles....Calc Phos
crawling sensation, with....Kali Phos
elderly, in....Calc Phos, Kali Phos
exertion, violent, after....Nat Mur
eyelids, irritated (see also Eyelids)....Nat Mur
feet....Kali Phos
hands....Kali Phos
insect bites, like....Nat Phos
inside of hands, soles of feet; thickest areas....Kali Phos, Calc Sulph
irritable areas of the skin may be sponged with a solution of the
   salts in tepid water and apply as needed....Nat Phos, Kali Phos,
   Mag Phos
ivy, or poison oak....Kali Sulph
legs....Kali Mur, Kali Phos
nervous irritation or pain, with....Kali Phos
nettles, as from....Calc Phos
pain, and; from 2:00 to 5:00 p.m.....Kali Phos
pain of nettle rash, and....Nat Mur
palms....Kali Phos
pruritus
   external auditory canal with scaly exfoliation....Kali Phos
   general, in....Calc Phos, Kali Phos
   palms and soles of the feet, of; no dermal pathology is
      present....Kali Phos
senile....Calc Phos
skin....Calc Phos, Silica, Kali Sulph, Kali Phos
soles....Kali Phos, Calc Sulph
toes....Nat Sulph
undressing, while....Nat Sulph
vagina....Calc Phos, Nat Phos, Kali Phos
violent; after physical exertion....Nat Mur
without eruptions....Calc Phos

JAUNDICE (see also Liver)
bitter taste, with, and constipation....Kali Mur
chill, caused by a....Kali Mur
diarrhea, with....Nat Phos
drowsiness, with....Nat Mur
gastric catarrh, caused by....Kali Sulph

gastritis, after....Kali Sulph
gastro-duodenal catarrh, caused by....Kali Mur, Nat Mur
primary remedy is Nat Sulph with the following....Kali Mur, Nat
   Mur, Kali Sulph
sluggish liver, with; give 12X potency three times/day....Kali Mur
vexation, after....Nat Sulph

## JOINTS

cracking....Nat Mur, Calc Fluor, Nat Phos, Nat Sulph
creaking....Nat Phos, Nat Mur
diseases
>  affecting the surface of....Calc Fluor
>  general, in....Ferr Phos, Silica
elbow
>  pain shooting through....Calc Phos
>  swollen....Calc Fluor
finger (see Finger, joints)
gouty enlargements of....Calc Phos, Calc Fluor
hip joint disease....Calc Sulph, Calc Phos, Ferr Phos, Silica, Kali
   Mur, Nat Mur
inflammation that has the appearance of a fungus....Kali Sulph
involvement in....Calc Fluor
knee inflammation (see also Knee)....Calc Fluor
pain
>  excruciating....Mag Phos
>  general, in....Kali Mur, Ferr Phos
>  violent....Kali Sulph, Calc Phos, Nat Mur, Mag Phos
rheumatism
>  chronic....Calc Phos, Nat Mur
>  general, in....Nat Phos, Calc Fluor, Silica
>  pain, violent....Nat Mur, Mag Phos, Kali Sulph, Calc
>     Phos
sore pain in....Nat Phos
swellings of and around joints; 6 tablets of each salt dissolved in
   hot water may be applied as a compress....Calc Fluor, Ferr
   Phos, Kali Mur
swollen, with fibrinous consolidation....Kali Mur
urticaria about joints....Nat Mur

## KIDNEY

disease....Calc Sulph, Nat Sulph
inflammation

general, in....Ferr Phos, Kali Mur, Nat Phos, Nat Mur
effects of....Kali Mur
nephritis, chronic....Nat Sulph
pains in....Ferr Phos, Calc Phos
stones....Calc Phos
urine, lithic deposits in....Nat Sulph

## KNEE (see also Joints)

anchylosis of....Silica
herpes in the bend of....Nat Mur
housemaids....Calc Phos, Silica
inflammation of, or knee joint....Calc Fluor
pain....Calc Phos, Nat Phos, Ferr Phos
soreness in bend of....Nat Mur
swelling of joint, hot, painful....Nat Mur
synovitis (see Synovitis)
weakness of....Nat Mur

## LABOR (see Pregnancy and Labor)

## LACTATION

encourages....Calc Phos, Nat Mur
lessens....Calc Fluor, Nat Sulph
loss of hair during....Nat Mur
nipples cracked and ulcerates easily....Silica
reduced from prolonged nursing....Calc Phos
salty and bluish milk....Calc Phos, Calc Fluor

## LACTIC ACID, excess; may result from too much sugar intake....Nat Phos

## LAMENESS

cold, from....Ferr Phos
paralytic....Kali Phos, Nat Mur
rheumatic....Kali Phos

## LANGUID, feelings associated with humid, oppressive weather....Nat Sulph, Nat Mur

## LARYNGITIS

dryness, with....Calc Fluor, Nat Mur
general, in....Ferr Phos, Kali Phos, Kali Mur, Nat Mur

## LARYNX

burning and soreness in....Ferr Phos, Calc Phos
closing by spasms or cramps....Mag Phos

irritated....Ferr Phos, Calc Fluor
painful....Ferr Phos
sore....Ferr Phos
tickling, with relaxed uvula....Calc Fluor, Nat Mur

LASCIVIOUSNESS....Calc Phos

LEAD POISONING, use 2X potency....Nat Sulph

LEGS (see also Extremities)
aches and pains with a feeling of heaviness; poor
    circulation....Calc Fluor
give way while walking....Nat Phos
itching of....Kali Mur, Kali Phos
jerking when at rest....Nat Mur
swelling, chronic....Kali Mur
weakness....Nat Mur, Nat Phos

LEUKORRHEA
acid....Nat Phos
acrid....Nat Sulph, Kali Phos, Silica
albuminous mucus....Calc Phos
corroding....Nat Sulph, Nat Mur
creamy
        general, in—-Nat Phos, Calc Phos
        yellow and watery....Nat Phos
egg white, like....Calc Phos
general, in....Calc Phos, Kali Mur
greenish....Kali Sulph
gushes, or flow is thick, creamy....Silica
honey-colored....Nat Phos
irritating
        general, in....Nat Mur, Mag Phos, Nat Sulph
        greenish-yellow....Nat Sulph
itching....Silica, Nat Mur
milky....Kali Mur
morning, worse....Calc Phos
orange-colored....Kali Phos
profuse....Silica, Kali Mur
prolonged bouts, after; acts as a constitutional tonic....Calc Phos
scalding....Nat Mur, Kali Phos
slimy....Kali Sulph
smarting....Nat Mur

sour-smelling....Nat Phos
thick
    bland discharge....Kali Mur
    offensive....Kali Phos
    white....Kali Mur
    yellow, purulent, sometimes blood-tinged....Calc Sulph
watery....Kali Sulph, Nat Mur, Nat Phos
white....Kali Mur
yellow....Kali Phos, Kali Sulph

LEUKEMIA....Nat Phos, Calc Phos, Kali Phos, Nat Sulph

LIGAMENTS, flaccidity of; uterine, rectal prolapses; uterine
    malpositions....Calc Fluor

LIGHT SENSITIVE (see Photophobia)

LIMBS (see Extremities, and the particular body parts)

LIPS
    burning, painful, cracked....Nat Mur
    chapped....Calc Fluor
    cold sores on; small ones....Nat Mur, Calc Fluor
    cracked....Calc Fluor, Silica, Nat Mur
    cracks are deep in middle of upper and/or lower lip or at corner
       of lips; painful....Nat Mur
    dryness of
       general, in....Kali Sulph
       lower lip, and skin pulls off in large flakes....Kali Phos
    heat in....Kali Sulph
    herpetic, hard....Calc Fluor
    hydroa-chronic inflammatory skin disease....Kali Phos, Nat Mur
    skin peeling off....Kali Sulph, Kali Phos
    sore on the inside....Calc Sulph
    swollen
       general, in....Nat Mur
       lower....Kali Sulph
       upper, painful....Calc Phos
    tumors on....Silica
    twitching, spasmodic....Mag Phos
    white....Kali Sulph

LIVER
    abscess about region of liver, painful....Calc Sulph

acidity, with....Ferr Phos, Nat Phos, Nat Sulph, Nat Mur

ailments; biliousness....Nat Sulph

biliousness, notably (see also Biliousness)....Nat Sulph, Calc Sulph

cirrhosis....Nat Sulph

congestion....Nat Sulph

disease, chronic....Mag Phos

disorders in the secretion and flow of bile....Nat Sulph

disturbances like biliousness, sick headache, nausea....Nat Sulph

dysfunction....Nat Sulph

engorged; worse lying on left side....Nat Sulph

faulty bile production and jaundice, associated with....Nat Phos

fever accompanies liver ailment....Ferr Phos, Nat Phos, Nat Mur, Nat Sulph

function, healthy, controls....Nat Sulph

general, in; important remedy for liver problems....Kali Mur

jaundice, with (see Jaundice)

pain

> cutting in region of liver....Nat Sulph
>
> general, in....Nat Mur, Kali Phos, Nat Sulph, Kali Mur, Calc Phos
>
> sharp, shooting....Nat Sulph

remedy, primary....Nat Sulph

sensitive....Nat Sulph

sluggish

> general, in....Nat Mur, Nat Sulph
>
> jaundice, with; give 12X three times a day....Kali Mur
>
> pale yellow evacuations, with....Kali Mur

sore to touch area....Nat Sulph

spots on skin....Kali Sulph, Calc Sulph

tongue white or gray (see also Tongue)....Kali Mur

torpidity....Kali Mur

trouble....Nat Sulph, Kali Mur

## LOCK JAW....Mag Phos

## LOWER BACK PAIN (see Back)

## LUBRICAN, anti-friction....Kali Sulph

## LUMBAGO

acid conditions, with....Nat Phos, Nat Sulph

dragging pain, with....Calc Fluor

early stages, during; inflammation and pain present....Ferr Phos

general, in....Nat Phos, Ferr Phos, Nat Mur, Calc Phos
pain on bending, severe; unable to straighten....Calc Phos
rheumatic pain in joints, cold or numb sensation....Calc Phos
strains, from; alternate with Ferr Phos....Calc Fluor, Calc Phos
worse cold and change of weather....Calc Phos

**LUNGS**
abscess of....Silica
congestion of....Ferr Phos
disease; third stage....Calc Sulph
edema of....Kali Phos, Nat Mur
inflamed....Kali Phos
soreness....Ferr Phos
wheezing, rales (see also Respiratory)....Kali Mur

**LUPUS OF THE SKIN**....Calc Phos, Kali Mur

**LYMPH NODES (see Glands)**

**LYMPHOID STRUCTURES,** enlargement of; tonsils, adenoids, cervical, axillary, inguinal and other glands (see also individual glands)....Calc Fluor

**MALABSORPTION (see Stomach, Digestion)** sip frequently; for water symptoms add a few tablets of Nat Mur....Ferr Phos, Nat Sulph

**MANIPULATION (see Subluxations)**

**MASTITIS**
discharge is brown and pus is offensive....Kali Phos
general, in....Calc Fluor, Silica, Calc Sulph, Kali Mur, Ferr Phos

**MASTOID PROCESS**
caries of....Silica
diseases of....Silica
pains below....Kali Sulph
periosteum diseased....Calc Fluor
swollen, sore....Ferr Phos

**MASTOIDITIS,** inflammation of the mastoid process; best results when dissolved in hot water, sipped....Ferr Phos, Calc Sulph, Kali Mur

**MASTURBATION**
children, in....Calc Phos
general, in....Calc Phos, Kali Phos, Silica

**MEASLES,** dissolve 6 tablets of each in a cup of hot water and sip a dessert spoonful every 2 hours; post-measles give Calc Phos and Kali Phos....Ferr Phos, Kali Mur, Kali Sulph, Silica

MEMORY (see Mental States)

MENINGITIS

general, in....Ferr Phos, Kali Mur

spinal....Nat Sulph

MENOPAUSE

abdomen has sensation of a weight or fullness....Kali Sulph

dizziness and hot flashes....Mag Phos

general, in....Ferr Phos, Kali Phos, Calc Phos, Nat Phos, Silica, Kali Sulph

hot flashes, helpful with; also sleeplessness, hot spells, and cold feet....Ferr Phos

palpitations, abnormal; pains....Mag Phos, Kali Phos

restlessness, nervousness, sensations of numbness, sinking sensations....Kali Phos

MENSTRUATION

absence of flow (see Amenorrhea)

acid symptoms, with; local irritation....Nat Phos

acrid....Nat Phos, Nat Sulph

anemia in young women....Calc Phos

black flow....Kali Mur

blackish-red flow....Kali Phos

blood is dark and clotted....Nat Phos, Kali Mur

bright red flow....Calc Phos, Ferr Phos

checked....Kali Mur

chilliness, with....Silica, Nat Sulph

clotted; dark clots with too frequent or too early flow....Kali Mur

coagulated, not....Kali Phos

cold extremities....Calc Phos, Ferr Phos

coldness, with; may be like ice....Silica

colic

general, in....Mag Phos, Nat Sulph, Kali Phos

nervous, sensitive females, in....Kali Phos

congestion, excessive....Ferr Phos

corrosive....Nat Sulph

constipation, with....Silica, Nat Sulph

cramps; give 3X for up to one week prior to menses, then 12X or 30X for one additional week....Mag Phos

dark flow....Mag Phos, Kali Mur, Calc Phos
dark, red flow....Kali Phos
delayed
        smarting discharges between periods with terrible
           sadness, especially during period; may occur with
           headache....Nat Mur
        young girls, in....Nat Mur, Kali Mur
diarrhea, morning, with....Nat Sulph
dysmenorrhea (see Dysmenorrhea)
early, too....Calc Phos, Mag Phos, Nat Phos, Kali Mur, Silica,
    Kali Phos
every two weeks....Calc Phos
every three weeks....Ferr Phos
excessive....Calc Phos, Kali Mur, Calc Fluor, Nat Sulph, Kali
    Phos, Ferr Phos
excitement and sleeplessness, with....Nat Phos, Kali Phos
fibrous....Mag Phos
flooding....Calc Fluor
flow too thick, excessive; accompanied by bearing down pains
    and flooding....Calc Fluor
flushed face, with....Calc Phos, Ferr Phos
foot sweats, fetid, with....Silica
frequent, too....Kali Mur, Calc Phos
fullness in abdomen, with....Kali Sulph
headache, with (see also Headache)
        after menses....Nat Mur
        associated with....Ferr Phos, Kali Phos
        before/during menses....Calc Sulph, Nat Mur, Kali Phos
        hunger, and....Kali Phos
        profuse flow with....Ferr Phos
hysteria, with....Kali Phos
icy coldness of body at commencement of flow....Silica
increased flow....Silica
irregular....Calc Phos, Ferr Phos, Kali Sulph, Kali Phos
lactation, during....Silica, Calc Phos
late, or delayed, from a cold; blood is dark and clotted....Kali
    Mur, Nat Phos
leukorrhea watery, with....Nat Mur
long lasting....Calc Sulph, Kali Mur
melancholy, with....Nat Mur
mental depression, with....Nat Mur

morning diarrhea, with....Nat Sulph

nervousness, with....Kali Phos

nosebleed before or during menses....Nat Sulph

odor, offensive or strong....Kali Phos

pain (see Dysmenorrhea)

pale color of the flow

        general, in....Nat Mur, Nat Phos

        women who are nervous and sensitive, in....Kali Phos

profuse....Kali Mur, Kali Phos, Calc Fluor, Nat Sulph, Ferr Phos, Nat Mur

prolonged; may cause anemia....Calc Phos, Kali Mur, Calc Sulph

retention of....Kali Phos

sadness before menses; may be excessive....Nat Mur

scanty flow....Kali Phos, Kali Sulph, Silica, Nat Mur, Calc Phos

sexual desire

        intense, after menses....Kali Phos

        preceded by sexual excitement....Calc Phos

spasmodic pains, cramps, labor-like/bearing down pain....Mag Phos

stringy and fibrous....Mag Phos

suppressed

        anemia, when arises from; faults in the diet....Calc Phos

        pill, after stopping; take along with Pulsatilla 3X in

            homeopathic potency....Calc Phos

        scanty, or, with full abdomen/yellow tongue....Kali Sulph

swelling of labia, with....Mag Phos

thin, watery blood....Nat Mur, Kali Phos

tough discharge....Kali Mur

twitching, with....Nat Mur, Calc Sulph

water retention, with; take before meals....Nat Sulph, Nat Mur

watery, thin discharge; depression of spirits and lassitude;

    morning headache....Nat Mur

weakness, great, with....Calc Sulph

weeping, with....Nat Mur

weight in abdomen, with....Kali Sulph

worse symptoms during menses....Nat Phos

MENTAL STATES, cell salts work best in the higher potencies for emotional issues

    aberrations....Kali Phos

    agitated....Silica

    agoraphobia-morbid dread of open spaces....Kali Phos

alone
>   likes to be....Ferr Phos, Nat Mur
>   wants to deal with their sorrow alone....Nat Mur

ambition, without....Calc Phos, Nat Phos

anger
>   easily; feels weak when anger has passed....Calc Sulph
>   irritability, with....Nat Mur
>   quickly, tendency to....Silica
>   trifles, at....Nat Phos

anxiety
>   future, about....Calc Phos
>   general, in....Kali Phos, Kali Mur, Nat Phos, Calc Phos
>   night, at....Nat Phos
>   restlessness, with....Kali Phos

anxious moods....Kali Phos

apprehensiveness....Nat Phos, Nat Mur, Kali Phos

attention, difficult to fix....Silica

awakens screaming....Kali Phos

awkwardness....Mag Phos

backwardness....Kali Phos

blushing from emotions....Kali Phos

brain and nerve tissues affected; when you need strength of mind
    or have an inferiority complex....Silica, Kali Phos

brain fog from overwork....Kali Phos, Nat Mur, Silica

carries things from place to place....Mag Phos

changeable moods....Calc Sulph, Kali Phos

change, during times of....Calc Phos

chattering of teeth, nervous....Kali Phos

cheerful excitement, better under....Kali Phos

children, in (see Children)

comprehension slow....Calc Phos

confusion
>   easily....Calc Sulph
>   general, in....Mag Phos, Kali Phos

consciousness, loss of, sudden....Calc Sulph

consolation, aggravated by....Nat Mur

contrary, sense of humor is becoming more....Kali Phos

conversation, disinclination to....Kali Phos

cretinism....Calc Phos

crossness in children....Kali Phos

cruel; if there's been cruelty to a partner or to child....Kali Phos

crying mood....Kali Phos
cries
        easily....Kali Phos
        tendency to....Mag Phos
dance and sing, inclination to....Nat Mur
dark forebodings; looks at the dark side of everything....Kali Phos
death, afraid of....Kali Phos
delirium
        general, in....Ferr Phos, Nat Mur, Kali Phos
        mutterings, low....Kali Phos
        talkative, very; being wide awake....Ferr Phos, Nat Mur
        tremors....Nat Mur, Kali Phos, Ferr Phos
        wandering mind....Nat Mur
dejection....Nat Mur
depression
        damp, chilly weather makes worse....Calc Fluor
        great....Calc Fluor
        mental or physical....Kali Phos
        mood depressed....Nat Mur, Kali Phos
        morning, worse, but cheerful in evening....Calc Sulph
        nervous....Kali Phos
        not sure why....Kali Phos
        primary remedy for depression....Kali Phos
        self-doubt, pressure, worry, during periods of....Kali Phos
        severe enough to keep a person from accomplishing the
            most simplistic task....Kali Phos
derangements
        general, in....Kali Phos
        head injury, from....Nat Sulph
despair
        getting well again, of....Nat Sulph
        long periods of time, for....Kali Phos
despondency
        business, about....Kali Phos
        change-of-life....Kali Phos
        generally....Kali Phos
        moods, of....Silica, Nat Mur, Nat Sulph, Kali Phos
determination, lack of....Silica
difficulty of thought....Silica
disappointment, after effects of....Calc Phos
discouraged

general, in....Silica, Nat Sulph, Ferr Phos
 depression and despondency feelings in the morning;
  have hard time getting started mornings....Nat Sulph
disgust of life....Silica
disheartened....Nat Sulph
disinclination
 conversation, to have....Kali Phos
 mix with people, to....Kali Phos
disposition to value money more than natural....Calc Fluor
dizziness (see Dizziness)
dread
 hot drinks, of....Kali Sulph
 nervous with no specific cause....Kali Phos
 noises, of....Kali Phos, Silica
dreams (see Dreams)
drowsiness
 feeling of....Mag Phos
 general, in....Nat Sulph, Nat Mur
 muscular weakness, with....Nat Mur
dullness
 feeling dull, not being able to concentrate....Mag Phos
 general, in....Kali Phos, Mag Phos, Nat Phos
dwells upon grievances....Kali Phos
emotional
 blushing from....Kali Phos
 hysteria, sudden....Kali Phos
 slow and plodding....Calc Phos
 violent emotions and ailments, corrects....Mag Phos
energy, want of (see also Vitality, Fatigue)....Kali Phos
excitement, excessive, banishes....Kali Phos, Silica
exhaustion
 extreme....Mag Phos, Silica, Kali Phos
 nervous
  colic, with....Nat Sulph
  general, in....Kali Phos, Mag Phos
  irritable, excited....Silica
express, inability to....Calc Fluor
fainting (see Faintness)
false impressions....Nat Phos, Kali Phos
fancies....Kali Phos
fatigues easily (see also Fatigue)....Ferr Phos, Nat Mur, Kali Phos

fear of

> burglars....Kali Phos
> falling....Kali Sulph
> financial ruin; groundless....Calc Fluor
> general, in....Kali Phos, Silica, Kali Mur
> groundless fears....Calc Fluor
> irrational....Kali Phos
> money troubles....Calc Fluor
> paralyzing, almost....Kali Phos
> thunder....Nat Mur
> suffers from terrible fears....Calc Sulph

fearfulness....Kali Sulph

feeble, becomes, when you need to think....Calc Sulph

fidgety feeling....Kali Phos

fingers clenched....Mag Phos

fits

> crying, of....Kali Phos
> laughing, of....Kali Phos

forgetfulness

> can't concentrate, and feeling dull....Mag Phos
> general, in....Kali Phos, Calc Phos

frazzled by job or life....Kali Phos

fretful....Calc Phos, Kali Phos

frequent episodes....Nat Mur, Kali Phos

fright, after effects of....Kali Phos

frolicsome....Nat Mur

fuzziness, suffering from....Nat Phos

giddiness, with gastric problems....Nat Phos

globus hystericus-a lump in throat during neuroses....Kali Phos

gloomy; everything looks horribly bleak....Kali Phos, Nat Mur

grief

> after effects of....Calc Phos, Kali Phos
> sorrow and despair for long periods of time....Kali Phos

grumpiness....Kali Phos

hallucinations....Kali Phos, Nat Phos

haunted by visions of the past....Kali Phos

hears footsteps on awakening at night....Nat Phos

homesickness, suffer from a vague feeling of....Kali Phos

homicidal impulses....Kali Phos

hopelessness

> future, about....Nat Phos, Ferr Phos

spirits low, with....Kali Phos, Nat Mur
hypochondriacal
    constipation, with....Nat Mur
    general, in....Kali Phos, Nat Phos, Nat Mur
hysteria
    debility, with....Nat Mur
    general, in; from sudden emotions; immediate effects by
        dissolving five tablets of each remedy in a small
        amount of hot water and sip....Kali Phos, Nat Mur
    obstinate....Silica
ill-humored
    children, in....Calc Phos, Kali Phos
    general, in....Silica, Kali Phos
illusions....Kali Phos, Mag Phos
imaginary objects, grasping at....Kali Phos
imagines
    furniture to be a person....Nat Phos
    starve, must....Kali Mur
impatience, great; nervousness....Kali Phos
indecisive about little things unimportant....Calc Fluor, Kali Phos
indifference
    everything, to....Ferr Phos
    finances, to....Kali Phos
    family, to....Kali Phos
    general, in....Ferr Phos
    surroundings, to your....Kali Phos
    yourself, to....Kali Phos
inferiority complex....Kali Phos, Silica
injuries to the head, from....Nat Sulph
insanity....Ferr Phos, Silica, Kali Phos
insulted easily....Calc Sulph
intense by nature; sensitive....Nat Mur
irritability
    easily, especially with yourself....Ferr Phos
    trifles, at, especially small noises....Nat Mur
irritation due to biliousness....Nat Sulph
lamenting....Mag Phos
lasciviousness....Calc Phos
laughter, excessive....Kali Phos
life has dealt many blows....Kali Phos
love; suffers from a love affair....Kali Phos

mania
>general, in....Ferr Phos, Kali Phos
>puerperal....Kali Phos

maniacal mood....Ferr Phos

melancholy
>general, in....Kali Phos, Nat Mur, Nat Sulph
>puberty, at....Nat Mur

memory
>impaired....Calc Phos, Kali Phos
>loss of, sudden....Calc Sulph
>names, decreased ability recalling....Ferr Phos
>plays tricks on you....Kali Phos
>poor
>>children, in; often thin, emaciated....Calc Phos
>>general, in....Calc Phos, Kali Phos, Mag Phos
>weak....Kali Phos

mental
>abstraction....Silica
>exercise, when excessive....Kali Phos
>worn-out....Nat Mur, Kali Phos, Silica

mind over-trained....Kali Phos, Silica

miserable....Calc Fluor

motionless, sits in stony silence; tired; may pace back and forth....Mag Phos

music
>aggravates....Nat Sulph
>emotions, increases feelings of....Nat Mur

nervous (see Nerves and Nervous States) breakdown....Kali Phos
>conditions, with symptoms such as nervousness, irritability, mental depression, sleeplessness....Kali Phos, Mag Phos
>exhaustion....Nat Phos, Kali Phos
>gets the best of you, and....Kali Phos
>dread, anxiety, fear, with....Kali Mur, Kali Phos
>irritability....Nat Phos
>jangled nerves....Kali Phos
>nerve nutrient; primary remedy....Kali Phos
>sensitivity increased....Kali Phos, Silica
>very, especially in lean people....Mag Phos

neurasthenia....Kali Phos, Mag Phos, Calc Phos, Nat Phos, Ferr Phos

night terrors in children....Kali Phos
noise
        over sensitive to....Kali Mur, Kali Phos, Silica
        startled at the least noise....Kali Mur, Kali Phos
nymphomania....Calc Phos, Silica, Calc Fluor
omits letters or words in writing....Kali Phos
order and direction, restores to mind and body....Kali Phos
outbursts, passionate....Nat Mur
overly sensitive....Silica, Kali Phos
over strained mentally....Kali Phos
over worked, the feeling of ....Kali Phos, Silica, Nat Mur
paces back and forth....Mag Phos
past visions, longs for; this haunts them....Kali Phos
peevish children....Calc Phos
personality
        changes....Mag Phos
        obstinate....Kali Sulph
problems, having trouble dealing with....Ferr Phos
pulsation, feeling of....Calc Sulph
rambling talk....Nat Mur, Kali Phos
restlessness....Nat Sulph
restraint, necessary for....Nat Sulph
sadness....Calc Fluor, Nat Mur
screaming....Kali Phos
sedative; especially if suffering from restless anxiety and almost
    paralyzing fears....Kali Phos
senility....Kali Phos
sensations
        ants crawling over body parts, of....Calc Phos
        ball in throat, of....Kali Phos
        insect bites, of....Nat Phos
        numbness, of....Nat Mur
        trembling, of....Kali Phos
senses, illusions of....Kali Phos, Mag Phos
sexual
        desire gone....Nat Phos, Kali Phos
        excess....Nat Phos
        increased desire....Mag Phos, Nat Mur, Nat Phos, Kali
          Phos
        persistent thoughts....Silica
shock; for immediate effects dissolve 5 of each in a little hot

water and sip frequently....Kali Phos, Nat Mur, Nat Sulph

shyness

        company, away from....Calc Sulph

        excessive, with blushing....Kali Phos

        general, in....Kali Phos

sighing

        general, in....Kali Phos, Nat Mur

        tendency to....Calc Phos, Nat Phos

sinking feeling internally; feel the need to eat to restore strength,
    or have a sense of exhaustion and nerve problems....Silica

sleepiness....Nat Mur

sleeplessness (see Insomnia)

sleep problems (see Sleep)

sluggish, from continued exertion/great emotional strain....Kali Phos

sociable, not feeling very....Nat Phos

solitude desired....Calc Phos

somnambulism-sleepwalking....Kali Phos, Silica, Nat Mur

sorrow; even for long periods of time....Kali Phos

spirits low....Calc Phos

startled at the least noise....Nat Mur

stupor; acute diseases....Nat Mur

suicidal tendency; when it takes total self-control to prevent
    taking one's own life....Nat Sulph

suspiciousness....Kali Phos

talks

        asleep, while....Kali Phos

        excessive....Ferr Phos, Nat Mur

        rambling....Kali Phos

        to self, constantly....Mag Phos

tempers

        bad in children....Calc Phos

        calms irritable tempers....Kali Phos

terrors at night in children....Kali Phos

think, the feeling that you can't; at a loss for words, or you
    hesitate and repeat yourself in a conversation; the feeling of
    "cobwebs of the brain"....Calc Fluor, Kali Phos

thought

        cannot concentrate....Calc Phos

        difficulty of....Silica

timidity....Kali Phos

tired of life....Silica, Kali Phos

tired feeling....Nat Sulph, Nat Phos, Kali Phos, Mag Phos, Nat
   Mur
trifles seem like mountains....Ferr Phos
unhappiness in life; those to whom life is not joyful....Kali Phos
unpleasant states, suffering from....Calc Phos
vexation, after effects of....Calc Phos
visions of past, haunted by....Kali Phos
wanders from one subject to another....Calc Phos
want of energy (see also Fatigue, Vitality)....Kali Phos
weariness....Kali Phos, Nat Mur
weeping
         disposition to....Kali Phos
         easily....Nat Mur
         excessive....Nat Mur
         sobbing, convulsive....Mag Phos
whining....Kali Phos
wildness....Nat Sulph
withdrawal; feel a need to withdraw from society....Kali Phos
words in writing or speaking are used wrong....Kali Phos
worry....Kali Phos, Nat Mur, Silica
yawning, hysterical....Kali Phos

## MIGRAINE (see Headache)

## MILK, BREAST (see Pregnancy and Labor, Nursing, Lactation)

## MISCARRIAGE (see Pregnancy and Labor)

## MOISTURE, excessive, in any part of the system....Nat Mur

## MORNING SICKNESS

general, in....Nat Mur, Nat Phos, Kali Phos, Kali Mur
pregnancy, during, with vomiting of sour fluids....Nat Mur
vomiting
         frothy, watery phlegm....Nat Mur
         sour masses, of....Nat Phos
         undigested food, of....Ferr Phos
         white phlegm....Kali Mur

## MOTION

aggravates symptoms
         after rest....Kali Phos
         general, in....Calc Phos, Kali Mur, Ferr Phos
ameliorates symptoms (makes symptoms better)

gentle motion....Kali Phos
walking in open air....Kali Sulph
brings on pain....Kali Mur

## MOTION SICKNESS (see Sea and Air Sickness)

## MOUTH

breath (see Breath)
canker sores (see Canker Sores, Mouth ulcers, Ulcerations))
coating, creamy, yellow at back part of roof of mouth....Nat Phos
cold sores (see Cold Sores)
cracked at the corners....Nat Mur
drooling....Nat Mur
dry, always; teeth deficient in enamel....Calc Fluor
dryness....Nat Mur
epithelioma....Kali Sulph
eruptions (see also Eruptions)
>    pimples and sore crusts around mouth....Kali Phos
>    vesicular (see also Vesicles)....Nat Sulph

excoriation of....Kali Mur
gums (see Gums)
gumboils (see Gumboils)
heat in....Kali Sulph
inflammation (see also Inflammation)
>    mucous membranes, of....Ferr Phos, Kali Mur
>    salivary glands, of, when excessive saliva....Nat Mur
>    stomatitis
>>        general, in....Kali Phos
>>        vesicular, caused by deposition of bile in
>>        mouth....Nat Sulph

mucus (see also Discharge, Expectoration, Catarrh)
>    eating, while....Calc Sulph
>    full of slimy mucus; mucus wells up in mouth....Nat
>    Sulph

noma....Kali Phos
ranula-cystic tumor....Nat Mur
rawness and redness of....Kali Mur
roof
>    soft palate has creamy yellow coating; also on
>    tongue....Nat Phos
>    sore to touch....Nat Sulph

saliva, clear watery, in fever....Nat Mur
salivation, excessive
       fever, with....Nat Mur
       general, in....Nat Mur, Kali Phos, Kali Mur
slime, full of; thick, tenacious, greenish-white; must cough
    up....Nat Sulph
sore....Nat Mur
taste (see Taste)
thrush (see Thrush)
trismus-tonic contraction of the muscles of mastication;
    lockjaw....Mag Phos
twitching at corners of the mouth....Mag Phos
ulcers (see also Ulcerations)
       aphthous ulcers
              borax use causes....Nat Sulph
              general, in....Kali Mur
              salivation, much, with....Nat Mur
              stress, from (see Mental States)
       ash-gray....Kali Phos
       corners, in....Silica
       general, in....Silica
       nursing mothers, in mouth of....Kali Mur
       palate, of....Silica
       perforating....Silica
       white; in children....Kali Mur
water gathers in....Kali Sulph, Nat Mur

## MUCUS (see Discharge, Expectoration, Catarrh)

## MUCOUS MEMBRANES

congested....Ferr Phos
dry....Silica
sticky, yellowish secretion, with (see also Secretion)....Kali Sulph
swollen....Silica

## MUMPS

convalescence, during; helps restore vitality....Calc Phos
fever; give while fever lasts; alternate with Kali Mur....Ferr Phos
general, in....Ferr Phos, Nat Mur, Kali Mur
hawking up of salty mucus....Nat Mur
lymphadenopathy and pain on swallowing; primary
    remedy....Kali Mur
salivation....Nat Mur

swelling of parotids....Kali Mur

## MUSCULAR CONDITIONS

extensors contracted....Nat Phos
general, in....Calc Fluor
hamstrings sore....Nat Phos
lockjaw....Mag Phos
movements, involuntary....Mag Phos
pains; aggravated by motion and relieved by heat....Ferr Phos
painful contraction of muscles....Nat Mur
relax, to....Mag Phos
relaxed in pelvic areas of females, after confinement....Calc Fluor
shaking of hands, involuntary....Mag Phos
strained (see Strained)
strength, failure of....Kali Phos
tremors....Mag Phos
twitching (see also Nerves)....Mag Phos
weakness....Calc Fluor, Kali Phos

## MUSCULAR SCLEROSIS....Nat Mur, Kali Phos, Silica

## NAILS

ailments of the nails, any....Silica
brittle....Silica, Calc Fluor
crippled....Silica
diseased....Kali Sulph, Silica
growth interrupted....Kali Sulph
hangnails....Nat Mur, Silica
ingrown toenails....Silica, Calc Fluor, Ferr Phos, Kali Mur
inward growing toenails....Silica, Kali Mur
pain
        roots, at....Calc Phos
        under....Nat Sulph
splitting....Silica
thin, brittle....Calc Phos, Silica
thick, crumbly....Calc Fluor, Nat Mur, Silica
ulcers around....Silica
white spots, with....Silica

## NASAL POLYP (see Polyps)

## NAUSEA

embrace, during and after....Silica
fatty food, after....Kali Mur

general, in....Nat Phos, Mag Phos, Kali Sulph, Nat Sulph

empty sensation in stomach, with....Kali Phos

immediately after a meal....Nat Mur

mornings....Nat Phos

morning sickness (see Morning Sickness)

sour risings, with....Nat Phos

vertigo, with....Calc Sulph

vomiting, and (see Vomiting)

## NECK

crick in....Nat Phos

emaciation of the neck in children....Nat Mur, Calc Phos

muscles feel weak....Nat Mur

nape, margin of hair with eruptions, itching....Nat Mur

stiff

> cold, from....Ferr Phos, Calc Phos
>
> general, in; add 6-8 tablets of each to hot water and soak a wide bandage in the solution and apply on the neck; renew every 3 hours....Ferr Phos, Nat Phos, Nat Mur

## NERVES AND NERVOUS STATES

ailments of; all phosphate cell salts are recommended for nerve ailments; phosphorus helps rebuild the nerves....Mag Phos, Calc Phos, Kali Phos

breakdown....Kali Phos

chills, nervous, with chattering of teeth, in fevers....Mag Phos, Kali Phos

chorea

> general, in....Nat Mur, Mag Phos, Kali Sulph
>
> stools retarded, with....Nat Sulph
>
> worms, from....Silica

clinched fingers or fists....Mag Phos

coldness, after attack of nervousness....Kali Phos

conditions with symptoms such as nervousness, irritability, depression, sleeplessness....Kali Phos, Mag Phos

debility

> nerve nutrient, especially motor nerves; for nerve pain, cramps and nervous twitching; helps to steady the nerves....Mag Phos
>
> nutritional tone, increases; improves blood quality; promotes assimilation of vital nutrients to the

nervous tissue....Calc Phos
>    primary cell salt; give in any illness of a nervous type;
>        when nerves are on edge; nerve nutrient....Kali Phos

exhaustion....Kali Phos, Nat Phos

fever of nervous origin....Kali Phos

insulator, acts as....Silica

jangled....Kali Phos

loss of
>    motor power....Kali Phos
>    sense of touch....Kali Phos

mental causes, from (see Mental States)

night, at....Ferr Phos

nutrient remedy for ailments of nervous character....Kali Phos

pain is felt keenly....Kali Phos

pain such as neuralgia, neuritis, sciatica and headache
>    accompanied by shooting, darting stabs of pain....Mag Phos

problems....Silica

shaking of hands, involuntary....Mag Phos

shootings along nerves....Nat Mur, Mag Phos

supply depleted, nervous....Kali Phos

thumbs drawn in....Mag Phos

tic douloureux....Ferr Phos, Mag Phos

tired feeling....Nat Mur, Nat Sulph, Nat Phos, Kali Phos, Mag
>    Phos

tonic for nerves....Nat Phos, Calc Phos, Mag Phos, Kali Phos

trembling
>    body, of the....Kali Phos, Calc Phos, Nat Phos, Nat
>        Sulph
>    limbs, of the....Calc Phos, Silica

tremors....Mag Phos

twitching
>    during sleep
>        hands, of....Nat Sulph, Mag Phos
>        feet, of....Nat Sulph
>    general, in....Calc Sulph, Mag Phos, Nat Mur
>    whole body during waking hours; relief quicker if given
>        in a little hot water....Mag Phos

weakness....Ferr Phos, Calc Fluor, Kali Phos, Calc Phos, Calc
>    Sulph

NETTLERASH (see Hives)

## NEURALGIA

acute pains, due to inflammation; alternate with Mag Phos....Ferr Phos

aggravates symptoms

    changes of weather....Calc Phos

    cold....Mag Phos

    cold weather....Nat Mur

    heat....Ferr Phos, Kali Sulph, Kali Phos

    hot, stuffy room....Kali Phos

ameliorates symptoms (makes symptoms better)

    gentle motion....Kali Phos

    open air....Kali Sulph

    pleasant excitement....Kali Phos

    warmth applied to area....Mag Phos

anywhere, with depression....Kali Phos

anus, of....Calc Phos

back pains....Mag Phos

bones aching, anemia, rheumatism, characterized by....Calc Phos

congestive, after taking cold....Ferr Phos

cramping, with; give when Mag Phos fails....Silica, Calc Phos

electric shocks, like....Mag Phos, Calc Phos

face and upper jaw regions, of....Mag Phos

failure of strength, with....Kali Phos

general pains; quick relief if given in hot water....Kali Phos, Mag Phos, Kali Sulph

heat, worse with; for acute pain dissolve 6 tablets of each in a cup of tepid water and sip frequently....Ferr Phos, Kali Sulph, Kali Phos

improves general health....Calc Phos

inflammation, for....Ferr Phos

intercostal....Mag Phos

melancholia, with....Kali Phos

nerve sheath tissues, helps....Silica

nervous persons, in; for depression, sleeplessness and irritability....Kali Phos

night, occurring at....Mag Phos, Calc Phos

nutritional tone of the nerves, improves....Kali Phos

obstinate

    heat or cold gives no relief....Silica

    general, in....Silica, Mag Phos, Calc Sulph

night, occurs at....Silica, Calc Phos
ovarian; better lying on painful side....Kali Sulph, Mag Phos, Nat
  Sulph
pains in any tissues....Mag Phos
periodic....Nat Mur, Mag Phos
primary remedy for neuralgic pains; especially common in face
  and head nerves....Mag Phos
recurring....Calc Phos, Nat Mur
saliva, with flow of....Nat Mur
sensitive to noise and light....Kali Phos
shifting pain....Kali Phos, Mag Phos, Kali Sulph
spasmodic
        pains, for....Mag Phos
        violent, with darting, short, intense pain....Mag Phos
tears, flow of, with....Nat Mur
worse
        alone, when....Kali Phos
        morning....Nat Mur, Ferr Phos
        night, at....Kali Phos
        outside, when....Mag Phos

NEURASTHENIA....Kali Phos, Mag Phos, Calc Phos, Nat Phos, Ferr Phos

NIGHTMARES, also treat cause....Kali Phos, Nat Phos, Nat Mur, Calc
Sulph, Calc Fluor

NIGHT SWEATS
general, in....Kali Sulph, Silica
profuse
        fever, with....Nat Mur, Calc Phos, Silica
        head and neck, around....Mag Phos, Calc Phos

NOISES (see Ears, noises)

NOSE
bone, nasal
        ailments of....Calc Fluor
        caries of....Silica
        diseased....Calc Fluor
        periosteum affected....Silica
        polyp, large and pedunculated....Calc Phos
bleeding-epistaxis
        afternoons....Kali Mur
        anemic people, in, with thin/watery blood....Nat Mur

blowing thick yellow crusts from nose, after....Kali Phos
bright red....Ferr Phos
children, in....Ferr Phos
coughing causes....Nat Mur
delicate constitutions; thin blood, blackish, or
    coagulating....Kali Phos
first remedy to give....Ferr Phos
menses, during or before....Nat Sulph
predisposition to....Kali Phos
stooping causes....Nat Mur
burning in....Nat Sulph
catarrh (see also Catarrh, Coryza, Discharge, Exudation)
    acute or chronic; slimy yellow-green discharge....Ferr
        Phos, Kali Sulph
    albuminous discharge, thick, tough, from the posterior
        nares causing constant hawking and expectoration;
        worse out of doors....Calc Phos
    anemic person, of....Nat Mur, Calc Phos
    chronic
        general, in....Nat Mur, Silica
        purulent discharge....Kali Sulph, Silica
        swollen, ulcerated; takes cold readily....Calc
        Phos, Kali Mur
    clear, watery....Nat Mur
    conditions; gargle or spray area....Nat Mur
    dry, with stuffy sensation....Kali Mur
    dryness and stiffness of nose; hawking of mucus from
        the back part of the throat; after a week follow with
        Calc Phos....Kali Mur
    evening, worse....Kali Sulph
    fetid discharge, with....Kali Phos
    fever, accompanied by....Ferr Phos
    fever, with; give after Ferr Phos to promote
        perspiration....Kali Sulph
    loss of taste and smell, with....Nat Mur
    morning, worse....Nat Mur
    naso-pharyngeal....Nat Phos
    old, with loss of smell....Nat Mur, Kali Sulph
    posterior nares, of....Nat Phos
    salty, watery mucus, with....Nat Mur
    slimy, yellow....Kali Sulph

slow to respond to other treatments....Kali Sulph
stuffy sensation in nose....Kali Mur
thick discharge from the nasal bones....Calc Fluor
trickling sensation....Ferr Phos
warm room aggravates....Kali Sulph
white, thick; not transparent....Kali Mur
cold....Calc Fluor
coldness at point of nose....Calc Phos
congested nasal mucous membrane....Ferr Phos
coryza (see Coryza)
crusts
    inside nose....Nat Mur, Silica
    offensive, yellow....Kali Phos
dryness
    loss of taste and smell, with....Nat Mur
    mucous membranes, of....Nat Sulph, Silica
    painful, with throat symptoms....Nat Mur
    posterior nares, of....Nat Mur
    scabbing, with....Silica, Nat Mur
edges of nostril
    boils, have....Silica
    inflamed....Silica
    itch....Silica
    sore....Calc Sulph
excoriations....Silica
growths, osseous....Calc Fluor
itching
    edges of nostrils....Silica
    general, in....Kali Sulph, Silica, Nat Phos
    tip, at....Silica, Nat Phos
    wings of nostrils....Nat Sulph
numb feeling on one side....Nat Mur
obstructed....Nat Sulph, Kali Sulph
odor offensive from nose....Calc Fluor, Nat Phos, Kali Phos
ozena, syphilitic....Nat Sulph
picking at....Nat Phos
pimples on nose (see also Pimples, Eruptions)....Nat Mur
redness
    itches, and....Silica, Kali Phos
    pimples, with....Nat Mur
rhinitis (see Rhinitis)

scabs in....Nat Mur, Kali Phos
scrofulous children, nasal affection in....Calc Phos
smarting in

> general, in....Mag Phos
> right nasal passage....Ferr Phos

smell, sense of

> decreased, with dryness and rawness of the
>   pharynx....Nat Mur
> loss or perverted; not connected to a cold....Silica, Kali
>   Sulph, Mag Phos, Nat Mur

soreness of....Calc Sulph, Calc Phos
sore, with small boils around edges of nostrils....Silica
stuffiness....Kali Sulph, Kali Mur, Calc Fluor, Nat Sulph
swollen

> general, in....Calc Phos
> scabs and scurfs in nose, with....Nat Mur
> scrofulous children, in....Calc Phos

ulcerated (see also Ulcerations)

> invertebrate....Kali Phos, Silica
> scrofulous people, in....Calc Phos

white around nose....Nat Phos

## NUMBNESS

creeping....Calc Phos
extremities, of....Nat Mur, Calc Phos, Kali Phos
feeling of; if parts are asleep alternate with Mag Phos....Calc Phos
general, in....Mag Phos, Calc Phos, Kali Phos

## NURSING

infant wants to all the time....Calc Phos
prolonged, after; acts as a constitutional tonic....Calc Phos
vomiting and diarrhea, milk causes; give to mother/baby....Silica
vomits immediately (see Vomiting)....Calc Phos, Silica, Ferr Phos

## NUTRITIONAL

aid; problems arising from malnutrition or poor diet....Calc Phos
defective....Calc Phos
general; one of the first to take if feeling run down....Calc Phos
problems; usually thin and weak looking, with possible allergy
   problems, plagued with cramps and nervousness; tend to have
   a dark complexion....Mag Phos

## NYMPHOMANIA....Silica, Calc Phos, Calc Fluor

OBESITY

    general, in....Nat Mur, Nat Phos, Calc Phos, Calc Fluor
    helps with assimilation of starches and fats in the meal; take 1
        hour before meals along with Calc Phos....Calc Fluor

ODORS, eliminates certain offensive body odors....Kali Phos

OPERATIONS (see Surgical Operations)

OSSEOUS (see Bones)

OTITIS (see Ears)

OVARIAN

    inflamed condition of the ovary
        chronic....Kali Phos, Calc Phos
        general, in....Ferr Phos, Kali Mur, Mag Phos
        pain, much....Mag Phos
        gonorrhea, from....Nat Phos, Kali Mur
    neuralgia
        general, in; better lying on painful side....Mag Phos, Nat
           Sulph, Kali Sulph
        pain radiating across lower back....Kali Phos

PAIN

    aching; seems to tear downward; almost paralyzing....Kali Phos
    ache, dull; take 3X potency every 20 minutes....Kali Mur
    acidity, associated with....Nat Phos
    acute
        aggravated by
           exertion....Kali Mur, Ferr Phos
           fatigue....Kali Phos
           motion....Ferr Phos, Kali Mur
           warmth of bed....Kali Mur
        general; dissolve 6 tablets in a cup of hot water and sip
           frequently; repeat as needed; pain has a stabbing,
           boring sensation....Mag Phos
    aggravates pain
        cold, or cold air....Kali Phos, Mag Phos
        eating, after....Calc Phos
        evenings....Kali Sulph
        heated, stuffy atmosphere; worse evenings....Kali Sulph
        motion....Ferr Phos, Kali Mur
        right side, on....Mag Phos

touch....Mag Phos
water, cold....Mag Phos
ameliorates pain
    bending double....Mag Phos
    cold....Ferr Phos, Kali Mur
    friction....Mag Phos
    heat or warmth....Mag Phos
    motion....Kali Sulph, Kali Phos
    open air—Kali Sulph
    pressure, from....Mag Phos
    walking in open air....Kali Sulph
back (see Back)
bearing down....Calc Fluor
bodily, felt too acutely....Kali Phos
boils, gumboils, abscesses, due to (see also Gumboils)....Silica
bones and joints with deep-seated pain; worse night; sensation of
    numbness or the trickling of cold water; better movement of
    limbs....Calc Phos
bones, of; worse standing....Calc Sulph
boring....Mag Phos
brain, base of; violent....Nat Sulph, Nat Phos
breast, of....Mag Phos, Kali Phos
burning sensation, with....Ferr Phos
cancer, of....Kali Phos
chest (see Chest)
chilblains (see Frostbite)
children growing, of....Ferr Phos
coccyx, in....Calc Phos, Nat Sulph, Silica
congestive....Ferr Phos, Kali Sulph
cramp-like....Mag Phos
cuts and wounds, from; apply powdered tablets topically....Ferr
    Phos
darting and intense; intermittently....Mag Phos
digestive; associated with acidity, heartburn, sour acid
    rising....Nat Phos
electrical shocks, like....Mag Phos, Calc Phos
evening, in....Kali Sulph
excruciating, violent and spasmodic as in arthritis....Mag Phos
extremities, of, due to poor circulation....Calc Fluor
eyes (see Eyes)
feet, through....Silica

finger nails (see Nails)
food, associated with (see Dyspepsia)
frostbite (see Frostbite)
gastric; after eating fatty or rich foods....Kali Mur
general
       felt acutely, if,,,,Kali Phos
       most common remedies for pain....Ferr Phos, Mag Phos
gout (see Gout)
growing pains in children....Ferr Phos
gums (see Gums)
head, in (see Headache)
heart (see Heart)
inflammatory (see Inflammation)
intercostal, neuralgic (see also Neuralgia)....Mag Phos
itching of the skin, with nervous irritation or crawling
   sensation....Kali Phos
joints, in (see Joints)
kidney, in....Calc Phos, Ferr Phos
knees, in....Calc Phos, Nat Phos, Ferr Phos
leg aches and pain; feeling of heaviness due to poor
   circulation....Calc Fluor, Calc Phos
lightning-like....Mag Phos, Kali Mur
limbs, of; aches and pains due to bad circulation....Calc Fluor
liver, in (see Liver)
localized; better with warmth applied; worse going outside....Mag
   Phos
low back (see Back)
menstrual (see Menstruation)
motion brings it on....Kali Mur, Ferr Phos
moves from place to place in the body; recurrent....Mag Phos
muscular and articular; aggravated by motion; relieved by
   heat....Ferr Phos
nettle rash itch, of....Nat Mur
neuralgic (see Neuralgia)
periodical....Kali Sulph
pressure
       better from....Mag Phos
       worse from....Ferr Phos, Kali Mur
rectum, in....Calc Phos, Mag Phos
relieved by warmth or heat....Mag Phos
restlessness, with....Mag Phos, Kali Phos

rheumatic
>    anywhere; worse moving; better from warmth....Ferr
>        Phos
>    general, in....Kali Sulph
>    joints, in....Nat Phos
>    motion, only with....Kali Mur
>    night, at, in bed....Kali Mur
>    rheumatism, of (see Rheumatism)
>    wandering in joints; inflammatory pains....Kali Sulph

rising, when....Kali Phos, Nat Mur
sacro-iliac synchondroses....Calc Phos
secretions watery, increased, with; examples are tears, nasal dis-
>    charge, urine, blisters, blebs on the skin....Nat Mur

sciatica (see also Sciatica)....Mag Phos
severe; worse at night....Calc Phos
sharp, sudden twinges....Mag Phos
shifting
>    fleeting; wandering rheumatic pains in the joints;
>        alternate with Ferr Phos in the treatment of
>        inflammatory pains....Kali Sulph
>    general, in....Calc Phos, Kali Sulph, Mag Phos

shin-bones, in....Calc Phos, Nat Phos
shooting....Mag Phos
side, stitches in....Ferr Phos
soles of feet....Nat Phos, Kali Phos
spasmodic, cramping....Mag Phos
spinal cord, of....Mag Phos
stomach (see Stomach)
strain, from (see Strains)
suppurations and festering conditions, due to....Silica
swellings, soft; accompanied by white fibrinous discharge;
>    tonsillitis with swelling of cheeks and gums....Kali Mur

throbbing, with heat, inflammation and congestion; can apply
>    powdered tablets topically....Ferr Phos

toothache (see Teeth)
trembling, with....Mag Phos
trickling of cold water, like....Calc Phos
twitching and fidgeting, with....Mag Phos
wandering....Kali Sulph, Mag Phos
worse
>    evenings....Kali Sulph

right side, on....Mag Phos
warm weather....Kali Sulph
wrist, of....Nat Phos

## PALATE

inflamed....Ferr Phos
sensitive....Nat Sulph
tickling; enlarged soft palate, from....Calc Fluor
ulcer on....Silica
yellow coating on....Nat Phos

## PALMS (see Hands)

## PALPITATIONS

anxiety, with....Calc Phos, Nat Mur
blood flow, excessive, from....Kali Mur
cardiac....Mag Phos
digestive causes, from....Nat Phos
emotions, from....Kali Phos
exertion, from....Kali Phos
inflammation, accompanied by....Ferr Phos
mental/emotional causes, from....Kali Phos
nervous causes, from....Mag Phos, Kali Phos
pulse
    felt in different parts of body....Nat Phos
    rapid....Ferr Phos
rheumatic fever, after....Kali Phos
sleeplessness, with....Kali Phos
spasmodic....Mag Phos
stairs, from going up....Kali Phos
violent motion, from....Silica, Ferr Phos

## PANCREATIC

disease....Calc Sulph, Calc Phos
weakness....Nat Sulph, Kali Mur, Nat Phos, Kali Phos

## PARALYTIC CONDITIONS

any part of body....Kali Phos, Nat Mur
atrophic....Kali Phos
bladder, of....Kali Phos
creeping....Kali Phos
facial....Kali Phos
general, in....Kali Phos
infantile....Kali Phos

lameness....Kali Phos, Nat Mur
locomotor....Kali Phos
paresis....Kali Phos
rheumatic....Kali Phos, Calc Phos, Ferr Phos
suddenly comes on....Kali Phos
tabes dorsalis, from....Silica
tendency to....Kali Phos

PAROXYSMS, dissolve in hot water to bring quicker relief....Mag Phos

PEMPHIGUS-SKIN DISEASE
general, in....Nat Sulph, Nat Mur, Silica
malignum....Kali Phos

PEP, lacks (see also Vitality)....Kali Phos

PERITONITIS
first stages when area is painful to the touch....Ferr Phos
general, in; dissolve 6 of each in a cup of hot water and sip
frequently....Ferr Phos, Kali Mur, Kali Sulph, Mag Phos

PERSPIRATION
acid....Nat Phos
chronic, fetid
axilla, of; feet....Silica
legs, on....Kali Mur
clammy, on body, with fever....Calc Phos
cold sweat, on face with fever....Calc Phos
daytime, excessive, with fever....Nat Mur
debilitates....Kali Phos
decreased....Silica
eating, while....Kali Phos, Nat Mur
excessive, with offensive smell, especially of the feet; bottom part
of the body has decreased sweating, with the upper body
sweating too much....Silica
exhausting, excessive, while eating; with fever....Kali Phos, Calc
Phos
fetid....Kali Phos
general, in....Mag Phos
head, about
general, in....Silica, Calc Phos
profuse and on neck....Mag Phos, Calc Phos
lack of....Kali Sulph
night sweats (see Night Sweats)

offensive on the feet and armpits....Silica
profuse....Kali Phos, Calc Phos, Mag Phos
promote, to; skin inactive; may be hot, dry and harsh; dissolve in
    hot water and sip frequently....Kali Sulph, Ferr Phos
sour smelling....Nat Phos
suppressed; restores activity of the skin....Silica
thirst, without....Nat Sulph
weakening, and sour smelling....Nat Mur, Nat Phos

PERTHE'S HIP....Calc Phos

PERTUSSIS....Kali Mur

PETECHIAE....Kali Phos

PHARYNX
abscess in (see Abscess)
adherent crusts in....Kali Mur
burning and soreness in....Calc Phos
dryness and rawness in....Nat Mur
exudate (see Exudation)
inflammation of....Kali Mur, Nat Mur
weary feeling in....Kali Sulph

PHLEBITIS, the first four may also be dissolved and used in a
    compress....Ferr Phos, Kali Mur, Nat Phos, Calc Fluor, Kali Phos

PHOTOPHOBIA
artificial light, sensitive to....Calc Phos, Mag Phos
great intolerance to light....Ferr Phos, Calc Phos

PHYSICAL, exertion tires you easily (see also Vitality, Fatigue)....Ferr Phos

PILES (see Hemorrhoids)

PIMPLES (see also Eruptions, Pus)
adolescence's face and shoulders; a cleansing of the blood is
    necessary to correct this condition....Silica, Calc Sulph
clear face, to
        general, in——Silica, Calc Sulph, Calc Phos, Kali Sulph
        discharge of pus, with; add to other indicated
            remedies....Kali Mur
face, full of
        general, in....Kali Phos, Nat Sulph, Silica, Calc Phos,
        Calc Sulph
        matter forms, if....Calc Sulph, Calc Phos

many little and matterless; under the hair that bleed when
  scratched; precede with Silica....Calc Sulph
matterly scabs on heads of pimples....Calc Sulph
nose, on....Nat Mur
puberty, at....Calc Phos, Calc Sulph
pustules (see Pustules)
tender under beard....Calc Sulph
vesicles, covered with....Nat Mur, Nat Sulph
white, thick matter, filled with; on face and neck, especially after
  errors in diet....Kali Mur

## PLEURISY

fibrinous effusion, with....Kali Mur
first stage of; after Ferr Phos give Kali Mur....Ferr Phos
general, in; dissolve in hot water; take in frequent sips....Ferr
  Phos, Kali Mur, Nat Mur

## PNEUMONIA, dissolve eight tablets of each in a cup of hot water and
sip frequently; repeat as needed; give Nat Mur occasionally if
there are watery symptoms....Ferr Phos, Kali Mur, Calc Phos,
Silica, Kali Sulph

## POISON OAK/IVY

general, in....Kali Sulph, Nat Mur
itching, for....Kali Sulph
vesicles, small, hard, from severe cases that form scabs; apply
  topically with a cotton swab by dissolving in water and
  applying to the lesion....Kali Sulph

## POLYPS

general, in....Calc Phos, Calc Fluor, Nat Mur, Kali Sulph
nasal; large and pedunculated....Calc Phos
soft....Kali Sulph

## POLYURIA (see Urine)

## POSITIONS, having trouble dealing with....Ferr Phos

## POTT'S DISEASE....Calc Phos

## PREGNANCY AND LABOR, symptoms of

abortion tendency (see Pregnancy, miscarriage)
after pains
          general, in....Kali Phos, Mag Phos
          weak, due to feeble contractions....Ferr Phos, Calc Fluor

agalactia-absence of milk secretion after childbirth....Nat Mur, Calc Phos

breast

>burning in....Calc Phos
>
>enlarged feeling....Calc Phos
>
>cancerous tumor of....Silica
>
>fistulous....Silica
>
>hard lumps in....Calc Fluor, Silica
>
>ulcers of....Silica

convulsions, puerperal....Mag Phos

cramps in leg....Mag Phos

decline

>childbirth, after....Calc Phos
>
>nursing, prolonged, from....Calc Phos
>
>pregnancy, during....Calc Phos

delivery, promotes normal; take in hot water; frequent sips....Kali Phos, Mag Phos

expulsive efforts, excessive....Mag Phos

feet

>pain, during pregnancy....Silica
>
>soreness and lameness....Silica

fever

>childbed....Kali Mur, Kali Phos
>
>puerperal....Kali Mur, Kali Phos

general, in; need final 3 months....Calc Phos, Kali Phos, Calc Fluor

hair loss during childbirth and lactation....Nat Mur

labor, eases; take in hot water in frequent sips....Kali Phos, Mag Phos

labor pains, spasmodic....Mag Phos

limbs, weariness in all, during pregnancy....Calc Phos

mania, puerperal....Kali Phos

mastitis; discharge is brown and pus offensive....Kali Phos

milk (see Lactation)

miscarriage

>tendency to abort....Silica
>
>term, not carrying to....Calc Phos
>
>threatened....Mag Phos, Kali Phos

morning sickness (see Morning Sickness)

nipples, crack and ulcerate easily....Silica

nursing (see Nursing)

pain

    false, ineffectual and tedious....Kali Phos

    feeble....Kali Phos

    feet, in, during pregnancy....Silica

    spasmodic....Mag Phos

Phlegmasia alba Dolens-acute edema....Nat Sulph

puerperal

    convulsions....Mag Phos

    fever....Kali Mur, Kali Phos

    mania....Kali Phos

urine, can't hold....Ferr Phos

vomiting (see also Vomiting)

    foods, of, which leave acid taste in mouth....Ferr Phos

    sour masses, of....Nat Phos

    undigested food, of....Ferr Phos

    watery, frothy phlegm, of....Nat Mur

    white phlegm, of....Kali Mur

## PREMATURE OLD AGE....Calc Phos, Kali Phos, Silica

## PROLAPSE

internal organs, of....Silica, Calc Fluor

sinking feeling, with....Nat Phos, Calc Phos

sitting relieves....Nat Mur

womb, of, with dragging pains....Calc Fluor

## PROSTATE PROBLEMS

enlargement....Calc Fluor, Kali Mur, Nat Sulph, Mag Phos

inflammation....Ferr Phos, Silica

discharge of fluid....Nat Mur, Calc Fluor

suppuration of prostate in prostatitis....Silica

## PROSTRATION....Kali Phos

## PROUD FLESH....Silica, Kali Mur, Calc Sulph

## PRURIGO, chronic skin condition marked by itchy papules on extensor surfaces of limbs....Calc Phos

## PRURITUS (see Itching)

## PSOAS, ABSCESS....Silica

## PSORIASIS

dry....Nat Mur

primary remedy; tablets can be dissolved in water and applied

directly to lesion with a cotton swab....Kali Sulph
vaginal....Calc Phos

PSYCHOLOGICAL PROBLEMS (see Mental States)

PULSATION, feeling of....Calc Sulph

PULSE
all over the body, felt....Nat Phos, Nat Mur
below normal....Kali Phos
different parts or the body, felt in....Nat Phos
full and round, not rope like....Ferr Phos
intermittent....Kali Phos, Nat Mur
irregular....Kali Phos, Nat Mur
quickened....Ferr Phos, Kali Sulph
rapid....Ferr Phos, Kali Sulph, Kali Phos, Nat Mur, Silica
scarcely perceptible....Kali Sulph
sluggish....Kali Phos, Kali Sulph
slow, feeble....Kali Phos, Kali Sulph, Ferr Phos
subnormal, in fever....Kali Phos

PUS (see also Discharge, Exudations)
discharging pus such as on the heads of pimples, pustules, or
suppurating scabs....Calc Sulph, Silica
formation or threatened suppuration such as abscesses, boils,
gumboils, styes; give in all pyrogenic formations that are
chronic....Silica
shortens suppurative process....Calc Sulph
white, in wounds....Silica

PUSTULES (see also Discharge, Pus, Exudations)
face....Calc Sulph, Kali Phos, Kali Mur
forehead, on....Nat Mur
general, in....Kali Mur, Silica, Calc Sulph, Kali Phos
malignant....Kali Phos, Silica
pimples (see Pimples)
vesicles, covered with....Nat Mur, Nat Sulph
watery....Nat Mur, Kali Mur

PUTRID STATES (see Cleanser)....Kali Phos

PYORRHEA; in stubborn cases take Calc Sulph instead of Nat
Phos....Kali Mur, Nat Phos, Calc Fluor, Silica

QUINSY (see also Tonsils)

  general; dissolve 6 tablets of each in a cup of hot water and sip a
   teaspoonful every hour; repeat as needed....Ferr Phos, Kali
   Mur, Nat Phos
  periodical....Silica
  pus discharged....Calc Sulph

RASH

  fungus (see Fungus)
  hives (see Hives)
  measles-like....Kali Sulph
  rose-colored....Nat Phos

RAYNAUD'S DISEASE....Ferr Phos, Nat Mur, Calc Phos

RECTUM (see also Anus)

  burning pain in....Nat Mur
  burns....Kali Phos
  fistula....Calc Phos
  itching....Calc Fluor, Nat Phos
  neuralgia in....Calc Phos
  pain in....Calc Phos, Mag Phos
  proctalgia-pain in or around rectum or anus....Nat Mur
  rawness....Nat Phos
  sphincter control, loss of....Calc Phos
  stitches in....Nat Mur
  stool, passing, painful....Mag Phos, Nat Mur
  weakness of....Kali Phos

RED BLOOD CELLS

  count abnormally low (see also Anemia)....Calc Phos
  decreased....Ferr Phos
  formation of red blood cells, helps in....Ferr Phos
  increases blood cells....Calc Phos

RESPIRATORY TROUBLES (see also Lungs)

  breathing difficult during damp weather (see also
   Breathing)....Nat Sulph
  colds, frequent, cough (see Colds, Cough)....Ferr Phos, Kali Mur

RESPIRATORY TRACT

  ailments, for the second stage of most....Kali Mur
  general, in....Nat Sulph
  inflammation

all conditions of....Ferr Phos

early stages, during....Ferr Phos

expectoration is yellow or green and slimy, when (see also Expectoration)....Kali Sulph

lungs (see Lungs)

symptoms, all, worse in damp or rainy weather....Nat Sulph

suffocates in heated room, and....Kali Sulph

RESTORATIVE powers after acute disease and infections....Calc Phos

RETCHING (see Vomiting)

RHEUMATIC ARTHRITIS (see also Arthritis, Extremities, Pain)

extremities, of, with crepitations; examples are in knees, ankles, feet, elbows, wrists, fingers....Nat Phos

finger joints, especially; urine dark red; pains go suddenly to the heart; sore hamstrings; helpful in hot, painful swellings of knee joints....Nat Mur

joints swelling, with; if fingers involved rule out Vitamin B6 or zinc deficiency....Nat Mur

lameness from....Kali Phos

pain (see Pain, rheumatic)

RHEUMATIC FEVER....Kali Mur, Ferr Phos

RHEUMATISM

acid-waste products, from build up in the blood of; associated with faulty elimination....Nat Phos

acute

articular-the connection of bones....Ferr Phos

fever, with; dissolve tablets in a cup of hot water and take teaspoonful every 2 hours....Ferr Phos, Nat Phos

first-aid; acute attacks; for pain, inflammation and congestion....Ferr Phos

aggravates condition

changes in weather....Calc Phos

damp weather....Nat Sulph

ameliorates condition (makes symptoms better)

gentle motion....Kali Phos

warmth....Ferr Phos

ankles, in....Calc Phos

articular-the connection of bones....Nat Phos, Calc Phos, Ferr Phos, Kali Mur

exertion, on....Kali Phos

fatigue, with....Kali Phos

general, in....Ferr Phos, Nat Phos, Silica, Nat Sulph

heat or cold, with....Calc Phos

inflammatory; acute or chronic cases; tongue yellow coated; other
acid symptoms involving the mouth and sweat glands; with
toxic and acid rheumatism. Silica and Kali Phos are also
recommended....Nat Phos

joints affected (see also Joints)....Nat Phos, Calc Fluor, Silica

morning, in....Kali Phos

motion, with....Ferr Phos, Kali Mur

muscular....Ferr Phos

night, at....Calc Phos

pain (see also Pain)

> better in open air....Kali Sulph
>
> cold, numb feeling, with; worse cold and changes of
> weather....Calc Phos
>
> gradually comes on....Ferr Phos, Mag Phos
>
> joints, in....Nat Phos, Calc Fluor, Silica
>
> shifting....Mag Phos, Kali Sulph
>
> stinging or shooting in toes....Calc Phos
>
> violent, in joints....Nat Mur, Mag Phos, Kali Sulph,
> Calc Phos
>
> wanders; severe; accompanied by a high fever....Kali
> Sulph

paretic condition of....Kali Phos

rheumatic conditions, and....Ferr Phos

soreness causes restless sleeping after 3:00 a.m.; worse getting up
and walking around....Kali Sulph

subacute....Ferr Phos

swelling

> joints, around....Kali Mur
>
> motion brings on pain; concerned with cases of
> inflammation, rheumatic or gouty pain and
> swelling....Kali Mur

toxic acid rheumatism....Nat Phos, Silica, Kali Phos

urates lodging around joints and muscles, breaks up....Silica

waste transport system of the body is dysfunctional; this
remedy removes the toxic poisons....Nat Sulph

toes, in, with stinging or shooting pains....Calc Phos

RHINITIS, initial stage of; may be accompanied by a watery, acrid discharge that excoriates the membranes (see also Nose)....Ferr Phos

RICKETS, primary remedy is Calc Phos....Calc Phos, Ferr Phos, Calc Fluor, Mag Phos

RINGING IN EARS (see Ears, noises)

RINGWORM

general, in....Nat Sulph, Kali Sulph, Calc Sulph, Nat Mur
primary remedy....Kali Sulph
scalp or beard, of....Kali Sulph

RISINGS (see Vomiting)

RUNDOWN CONDITION (see Vitality, Debility)

SACRO-ILIAC SYNCHONDROSIS (see Back, pain)

SALIVA (see Mouth)

SALT, excessive use of; salts food before tasting it....Nat Mur

SCALDS (see Burns)

SCALP

cold feeling on....Calc Phos
cradle cap....Kali Sulph, Kali Mur
crust, yellow....Calc Sulph
dandruff (see Dandruff)
eruptions (see also Eruptions)

> general, in....Kali Mur, Kali Sulph, Ferr Phos, Silica
> itching
>
> > margin of hair, on....Nat Mur
> > pustules, of....Silica
>
> margin of hair at the nape, on....Nat Mur
> moist....Kali Sulph
> nodules, with hair falling out....Silica
> occiput, on, offensive....Silica
> watery contents, with....Nat Mur
> yellow, thin matter, of....Kali Sulph

excrescences on....Calc Fluor
hair falling out (see Alopecia)
inflammation of scalp....Ferr Phos
itches....Calc Phos, Kali Phos
lumps on....Silica
nodules on....Silica
pain, excruciating, in head (see also Head, pain)....Mag Phos

painful pustules on....Silica
rough feeling....Mag Phos
scales on....Nat Mur, Kali Mur
scaling
    copious....Kali Sulph
    moist and sticky....Kali Sulph
    white....Nat Mur, Kali Sulph, Kali Mur
sensitive
    cold and touch, to....Ferr Phos
    general, in....Nat Sulph, Silica
soreness....Calc Phos, Ferr Phos
sore to touch....Ferr Phos, Silica
suppuration (see also Suppuration)
    callous edges, with....Calc Fluor
    scrofulous ulcers....Calc Phos
    yellow and purulent discharge, with....Calc Sulph
tight sensation of....Calc Phos
tumors on....Calc Fluor

**SCAPULA,** ache between (see also Back, pain)....Kali Phos, Calc Phos

## SCARLET FEVER

drowsy; give every 3 hours....Nat Mur
general, in; dissolve a tablet of each in a cup of hot water and give a teaspoon every hour until fever subsides; give liquid warm....Ferr Phos, Kali Mur, Kali Sulph, Nat Mur, Nat Sulph, Kali Phos
weak and sore throat, with; Kali Phos may be helpful....Ferr Phos, Kali Mur
skin, shedding of; give every 2 hours....Kali Sulph

## SCIATICA

chronic; if Silica fails give Calc Sulph....Silica
getting up from sitting, or turning in bed makes pain worse; no relief from any position....Nat Sulph
pain from....Mag Phos, Ferr Phos
primary remedy for pain and inflammation; take every 1/2 hour during acute attack....Ferr Phos
restlessness, when associated with sciatica; alternate with Mag Phos....Kali Phos
spasmodic pain, for....Mag Phos
warmth, better with; add to other indicated remedies....Mag Phos

SCROFULOUS CONDITION....Calc Phos, Nat Phos, Silica

SCURVY....Kali Phos, Nat Mur, Nat Phos, Calc Sulph, Kali Mur

SEA AND AIR SICKNESS; take Kali Phos and Nat Mur before
 departure then Kali Phos and Nat Mur at intervals during the
 trip; Nat Phos before meals is also helpful, especially
 when taken with a little lemon juice; take in hot water, if
 possible....Kali Phos, Nat Mur, Nat Phos

SECRETIONS
 albuminous....Calc Phos
 bloody and purulent....Calc Sulph
 bland....Calc Phos
 fetid....Calc Fluor, Kali Mur, Silica
 fibrinous....Kali Mur
 greenish....Kali Sulph
 honey-colored....Nat Phos
 irritating....Nat Sulph, Kali Phos, Nat Mur
 lumpy....Calc Fluor
 offensive....Kali Phos
 purulent....Kali Sulph, Calc Sulph
 serous....Nat Mur
 septic....Kali Phos
 sticky....Kali Sulph
 yellow
  general, in....Kali Sulph
  watery, and....Nat Sulph, Kali Sulph, Nat Mur
 watery....Nat Sulph, Nat Mur

SENILITY (see Aging)

SENSITIVE TO, overly
 cold air....Silica
 heat and cold....Calc Sulph
 heat and light....Nat Mur
 noise and light....Kali Phos, Silica

SEPSIS
 chronic, where poisons enter the bloodstream, due to the absorption of pathogenic bacteria from the infected area; can
  occur from the result of alcohol or disease (see also
  Cleanser)....Silica, Kali Phos

L DESIRE HAS CHANGED (see Desires, Mental States)

## SEXUAL ORGANS, FEMALE (see also Female Disorders)

dragging sensation in groin....Calc Fluor
external parts
>> inflamed and swollen....Nat Sulph
>> pulsation of; throbbing; tingling....Calc Phos
>> voluptuous feeling in....Calc Phos
>> swelling....Mag Phos
genital weakness and sexual neurasthenia....Calc Phos, Kali Phos, Nat Phos, Kali Sulph, Silica
groin pain throughout right side....Nat Phos
hair loss from pubic area....Nat Mur
labia, abscess of....Silica
menstruation (see Menstruation)
oophoritis (see Ovarian)
ovarian (see Ovarian)
pressing sensation toward genitals in the morning....Nat Mur
prolapse of one or more of the internal organs....Silica, Calc Fluor
sterility, general; also treat constitutionally....Kali Phos, Calc Phos, Nat Mur, Nat Phos, Silica
uterus (see Uterus)
vulva
>> inflammation
>>>> general, in....Nat Mur, Nat Sulph
>>>> vesicular....Nat Sulph, Nat Mur
>> itching
>>>> general, in....Nat Mur, Silica
>>>> pronounced....Nat Sulph
>> relaxed....Nat Mur
>> vagina (see Vaginal)

## SEXUAL ORGANS, MALE

balanitis....Kali Phos, Kali Sulph
coitus, prostration or weak vision after....Kali Phos
discharge of prostatic fluid....Nat Mur
edema
>> preputial....Nat Sulph
>> scrotal....Nat Mur, Nat Sulph, Calc Phos
emissions
>> chilliness, with....Nat Mur
>> dreams, without, during sleep....Nat Mur

nightly....Silica, Nat Phos, Kali Phos

  stool, during....Nat Mur

epididymitis....Ferr Phos

erethism, sexual....Silica, Nat Phos

external parts

  drawing in of testicles and spermatic cord    Nat Phos

  erections....Kali Phos

  itching....Nat Sulph

  voluptuous feelings in....Calc Phos

genital weakness and sexual neurasthenia....Calc Phos, Nat Phos, Kali Phos, Kali Sulph, Silica

groin

  dragging sensation in....Calc Fluor

  pain through right side....Nat Phos

hair loss from pubis....Nat Mur

impotence....Nat Mur, Kali Phos

induration of testicles....Calc Fluor

infertility....Calc Sulph, Kali Phos, Calc Phos, Nat Mur, Nat Phos, Silica

orchitis

  general, in....Kali Mur, Calc Phos, Ferr Phos

  suppressed gonorrhea, from....Kali Mur, Kali Sulph

prostatitis (see Prostate Problems)

scrotum

  itching....Nat Mur, Silica, Calc Phos, Nat Phos

  sweating of....Silica

spermatic cord, painful....Nat Mur

sterility, general; also treat constitutionally....Kali Phos, Calc Phos, Nat Mur, Nat Phos, Silica

testicles

  aching in....Nat Mur

  indurated, hard....Calc Fluor

  pain in....Ferr Phos

  swelling in....Nat Mur, Calc Phos

varicocele....Ferr Phos

## SHAKING OF HANDS (see Hands)

## SHINGLES

first stage of inflammation, heat, burning, pain; apply also in powdered form as a compress to the area....Nat Mur, Kali Mur, Ferr Phos

general, in; if worse from cold take Mag Phos instead of Ferr
Phos; better if taken in hot water; take Nat Phos before meals
if acidity is present....Ferr Phos, Kali Mur, Nat Mur
nervous symptoms, with....Kali Phos
pain, for; also apply powder topically to area in a compress....Ferr
Phos
second stage of inflammatory condition....Kali Mur
white, thick eruptions; may have a white-coated tongue and
light-colored stools....Nat Mur, Kali Mur

SHOCK (see First Aid, Injuries, Accidents)

SHOULDERS (see Back)

SIGHING (see Mental States)

SINUS

discharge (see also Discharge, Exudation, Catarrh)
clear, watery, causes soreness; mucus tastes salty....Nat
Mur
fibrinous....Kali Mur
purulent; the bone affected alternate with Calc
Fluor....Silica, Calc Sulph
raw egg white, looks like....Calc Phos
sticky, yellow or greenish....Kali Sulph
thin watery....Nat Mur
yellow and/or green....Kali Sulph
white
general, in—Calc Phos
fibrinous....Kali Mur
yellow, lumpy, affecting the bones....Silica, Calc Fluor
general, in....Silica, Calc Fluor, Calc Sulph
inflammation; alternate with indicated remedy for the
discharge....Ferr Phos
sinusitis, with thin watery nasal discharge....Nat Mur

SKIN

abscess (see Abscess)
ailments
bilious symptoms, with....Nat Sulph
facial eruption that contain albuminous fluid, especially,
with yellow-white scabs (see also Eruptions,
Pimples)....Calc Phos
blebs....Nat Mur, Nat Sulph, Kali Phos

bleeds when scratched....Calc Sulph
blisters (see Blisters)
boils (see Boils)
builds new skin, helps....Kali Sulph
burning
>dry, hot; lack of perspiration,...Kali Sulph
>itching hands, and....Kali Sulph
>sensation of burning in skin....Silica
burns, small....Kali Mur, Calc Sulph, Nat Sulph
cancer (see Cancer)
chapped, cracks, fissures in the palm; can be used externally
together with a skin salve after washing affected area
well....Calc Fluor, Calc Sulph
children; keeps skin healthy during illness....Kali Sulph
chronic skin diseases....Nat Mur
cold and clammy....Calc Phos
coldness of the limbs....Calc Phos, Nat Mur
complexion (see Complexion)
cracked and chapped
>general, in....Calc Fluor, Nat Mur, Silica
>palms, in....Calc Fluor, Calc Sulph
>toes, between....Nat Mur
crawling, stinging sensation....Kali Sulph, Kali Phos
creeping sensation....Calc Phos
crust, dry, becomes scaly....Kali Sulph
cuts, slow to heal (see also Cuts)....Calc Sulph
dermatitis
>dermatitis herpetiformis....Kali Phos, Nat Mur
>general, in....Ferr Phos, Kali Sulph, Kali Mur, Silica
dermatoses (see Dermatoses)
desquamation, to promote....Kali Sulph
dirty appearance....Nat Mur
discharge (see Discharge, Exudate)
discoloration
>copper-colored spots....Calc Phos
>freckles....Calc Phos
diseases
>builds new skin cells where there has been damage to
the old ones; if indicated, a remedy for emotional
state is used at the same time....Kali Sulph
>chronic....Nat Mur

general, in....Calc Fluor
disorders of the young and teen-agers; no vent to the surface for the pus of an unopened boil or pimple without a head; be sure to precede Calc Sulph with Silica; Silica will open a vent to the surface; Calc Sulph will assist in removing the pus; the condition may look worse as the pus vents, but this is the first step in healing....Calc Sulph
dryness
    excessive....Nat Mur
    general, in....Kali Sulph, Calc Phos
eczema (see Eczema)
edematous inflammation....Nat Sulph
eliminates waste materials....Calc Sulph
eruptions (see Eruptions)
erysipelas (see Erysipelas)
excoriations....Calc Phos
excrescences, sycotic....Nat Sulph
exudations (see Exudation)
fissures (see Fissures)
flaccid, torpid....Nat Mur
formation of new skin, aids....Kali Sulph
greasy, especially in areas with many sweat glands....Nat Mur, Kali Phos
hard, thickened....Calc Fluor
harsh....Kali Sulph
heals with difficulty....Silica
healthy, important to keep; lubricating agent; helpful in older people who tend to lose the lubrication in their skin....Kali Sulph
herpes (see Herpes)
horny skin....Calc Fluor
hot, dry....Ferr Phos, Kali Sulph
inactive; to promote perspiration (see also Perspiration)....Kali Sulph
inflamed (see Inflammation)
injuries (see Injuries)
irritating skin ailments; shingles (see also Shingles)....Kali Phos, Kali Mur
irritation, great....Kali Phos
itching (see Itching)
jaundice (see Jaundice)

liver spots....Calc Sulph, Kali Sulph

lubrication; helpful in older people who tend to lose it....Kali Sulph

main remedy for skin problems....Silica

maintains healthy skin....Calc Phos

moist scabs on skin; skin affections....Nat Sulph

nervous origins, conditions of....Kali Phos

nodes on skin....Calc Fluor

numbness (see Numbness)

pallid anemic appearance (see Complexion)

peeling, with or without sticky secretions....Kali Sulph

perspiration is suppressed (see also Perspiration)....Silica

pimples (see Pimples)

prurigo is chronic skin condition marked by itchy papules on extensor surfaces of limbs....Calc Phos

psoriasis (see Psoriasis)

pustules (see Pustules)

rash (see Hives, Rash)

rawness of skin in little children....Nat Phos

rubbing skin makes symptoms better....Kali Phos

scabs

>    general, in....Calc Phos, Kali Phos
>
>    golden-yellow....Nat Phos
>
>    moist....Nat Sulph
>
>    white....Calc Phos
>
>    yellow....Calc Phos, Calc Sulph

scalds, when suppurating....Calc Sulph

scales

>    dry crusts, from....Kali Sulph
>
>    eruptions scaling....Calc Phos, Kali Sulph
>
>    freely on a sticky base....Kali Sulph
>
>    general, in....Kali Sulph, Nat Sulph, Nat Mur, Kali Mur
>
>    greasy....Kali Phos
>
>    scalp, on (see also Scalp)....Nat Mur, Kali Mur
>
>    thin whitish; chief remedy....Nat Mur
>
>    yellow....Nat Sulph

secretions (see Secretions)

sensitive....Silica

shingles (see Shingles)

sore....Nat Mur

sores, slow to heal....Calc Sulph

soreness in bends of knees and elbows....Nat Mur
spring, every, the same skin symptoms return....Nat Sulph
spots
      coppery....Silica
      liver....Calc Sulph, Kali Sulph
suppuration (see Suppuration)
swelling (see Swellings)
tingling....Kali Sulph
tubercles, on....Calc Phos
ulcerations (see Ulcerations)
unhealthy, with inflammation tending to generate pus; problems
    such as skin diseases; cracked skin; skin itchy, dry and brittle;
    hand chapped; helps skin eliminate waste....Silica
vesicles (see Vesicles)
wrinkled, withered....Kali Phos, Calc Phos
worse symptoms in the evening, and in hot stuffy
    atmosphere....Kali Sulph

## SLEEP

awakens screaming....Kali Phos
awakened from pains or flatulence....Nat Sulph
better during sleep, symptoms....Nat Sulph
desires
      constant sleep....Nat Mur
      morning, in....Kali Phos, Nat Mur
drawing pain in the back, at night, during sleep....Nat Mur
dreams (see Dreams)
excessive....Nat Mur
falls asleep while sitting....Nat Phos
grinds teeth (see Teeth, grinding)
hard to awaken in the morning....Calc Phos
insomnia (see Insomnia)
jerking of limbs during sleep....Silica, Mag Phos, Nat Mur, Nat
    Sulph
restlessness
      excitement, from....Kali Phos
      exhaustion, from....Mag Phos
      general, in....Nat Phos
      hyperemia, from....Ferr Phos
      itching, from....Nat Phos
      nervous irritation....Nat Mur

worms, from....Ferr Phos, Nat Phos

worry, after....Kali Phos

screams during sleep....Nat Phos

sleeplessness (see Insomnia)

sleepwalking....Nat Mur, Kali Phos, Silica

sleepiness....Nat Mur

sleepy during day, wakeful at night....Calc Sulph

startled at the least noise during sleep....Nat Mur, Nat Sulph

stretching, excessive, on awakening....Kali Phos, Calc Phos

tired in the morning; unrefreshing sleep....Nat Mur, Nat Sulph

twitching of muscles on falling asleep....Kali Phos

wakeful at night....Calc Sulph, Kali Phos, Ferr Phos

wakes easily....Kali Phos

yawning, much (see also Yawning)....Silica

SLUGGISH CONDITION....Kali Mur

SMELL, loss of or perverted....Nat Mur, Silica, Kali Phos, Kali Sulph, Mag Phos

SNEEZING

colds, with; discharge is clear, watery, transparent mucus....Nat Mur

frequent....Nat Mur, Silica

general, in....Silica, Ferr Phos, Calc Phos, Nat Mur

ineffectual desire for....Calc Fluor

slightest exposure, from....Kali Phos

SPASMS

chronic conditions; chief remedy....Mag Phos, Kali Mur, Calc Phos

muscles, intestines, retinas, blood vessels, affecting....Mag Phos

general, in....Mag Phos, Calc Phos

night, at....Calc Phos, Silica, Mag Phos

painful....Mag Phos

provocation slight, from....Silica

relief quicker if given with a little hot water....Mag Phos

solar plexus, spreads from....Silica

tetanic....Mag Phos, Nat Mur, Calc Phos

vaginal area, constrictive spasms in....Mag Phos

SPEECH

difficult....Nat Phos

fatigues....Kali Sulph

nasal, slow....Kali Phos
slow in learning....Nat Mur
slow and inarticulate....Kali Phos
slowly speaks....Mag Phos, Kali Phos
spasms of stammering, or tendency to....Mag Phos

SPERMATORRHEA (see Sexual Organs, Male)

SPHINCTER CONTROL, loss of....Calc Phos

SPINAL BIFIDA
general, in....Calc Phos, Ferr Phos, Silica, Calc Fluor
ventosa....Calc Fluor

SPINE
anemia
    cord, softening of....Kali Phos
    general, in....Kali Phos, Nat Phos, Nat Mur
cord, pain in....Mag Phos
curvature
    helps with healing....Calc Phos
    sitting up is difficult....Calc Sulph
idiopathic softening of spinal cord....Kali Phos
irritation....Silica, Calc Fluor, Kali Phos, Nat Mur
overly sensitive....Silica, Nat Mur
soreness, up and down....Nat Sulph

SPLEEN
enlargement....Calc Fluor, Nat Mur
inflammation....Ferr Phos, Kali Mur, Nat Sulph
pain in....Nat Mur, Kali Phos
trouble....Kali Phos

SPRAINS
first aid remedy....Ferr Phos
muscular, if (see Strains)
pain of....Mag Phos
shock and after-effects of....Nat Sulph
spasm, with....Mag Phos
suppuration, with....Calc Sulph
swelling, with....Ferr Phos, Kali Mur
tendons and ligaments; make compress from these salts dissolved
in tepid water and applied to area....Calc Fluor, Ferr Phos, Mag
Phos, Kali Mur

STAMMER (see Speech)

STERILITY

general, in; also treat constitutionally....Kali Phos, Calc Phos, Nat Mur, Nat Phos, Silica

STIFFNESS

body, of the....Kali Phos, Nat Mur
cold, after....Ferr Phos
general....Mag Phos, Kali Phos
neck (see Neck)
rest, after....Kali Phos
swelling, with, due to uric acid deposits....Nat Phos

STIMULANTS, after effects of alcohol....Nat Mur

STINGS (see Bites)

STOMACH

abrasions, gastric....Nat Phos
ache

acidity of stomach, from....Nat Phos
bending double, better from....Mag Phos
chill, from....Ferr Phos
constipation, accompanied by....Kali Mur
eating relieves....Kali Phos
exhaustion, with....Kali Phos
flatulence, with....Mag Phos, Nat Sulph
food aggravates....Calc Phos
fright or excitement, from....Kali Phos
loose stools, with....Ferr Phos
melancholia, with....Kali Phos
pain and salivation, with....Nat Mur
pressure aggravates....Ferr Phos
warmth, better from....Mag Phos
worms, accompanied by....Nat Phos

all conditions when there is sour, acid risings, or tongue is moist with creamy yellow coating....Nat Phos
appetite (see Appetite)
bloated feeling....Calc Phos
burning heat in....Calc Sulph, Kali Sulph, Calc Phos, Ferr Phos
catarrh, with yellow, slimy coated tongue; chronic....Kali Sulph
cramps....Mag Phos

deathly sickness at stomach....Ferr Phos
dilation of....Mag Phos, Calc Fluor, Nat Phos, Kali Phos, Nat
    Sulph
disturbances; important remedy....Calc Phos
dyspepsia (see also Dyspepsia, Gastric Disturbances)
        belching, with (see Eructations)
        flatulence, with (see also Flatulence)
empty feeling in....Nat Phos
enlargement....Mag Phos, Kali Phos
eructations-belching (see Eructations)
faint, sick feeling in stomach region....Calc Phos
faintness at....Kali Sulph
fatty and rich foods make symptoms worse....Kali Mur
fluids, frothy, sour, feel full of....Nat Phos
food aggravates
        distress from food....Calc Phos
        general, in....Calc Phos
        lying in a lump, seems to be....Calc Phos
        pain, causes....Nat Phos
        vomiting, causes....Ferr Phos
fullness and pressure in....Kali Sulph
gas (see Flatulence)
gnawing, empty feeling, even after eating....Calc Phos
hawking, constant, of foul slimy mucus from stomach....Nat
    Sulph
heat feeling in stomach....Nat Phos, Kali Sulph
heaviness in....Nat Sulph, Calc Phos
hemorrhage from stomach....Kali Mur, Ferr Phos
hungry (see Appetite)
indigestion (see Dyspepsia, Digestion, Gastric Disturbances)
induration of pylorus....Silica
intolerance of stimulants....Silica
malabsorption/malassimilation
        aids in assimilation....Calc Phos, Silica, Nat Phos
        fats, of....Nat Phos
        general, in....Kali Sulph, Calc Phos
        hydrochloric acid production, helps in....Kali Mur, Nat
        Mur
        intestinal....Mag Phos
        prevents malabsorption of nutritional elements....Silica,
        Nat Phos

mucus welling up in....Nat Sulph
neuralgia of....Mag Phos

pain
        abdominal ring, in....Nat Mur
        belching relieves sometimes....Calc Phos
        colicky....Kali Sulph, Kali Sulph, Mag Sulph
        constant, in pit of stomach....Kali Phos
        deep-seated....Kali Sulph
        eating
                after....Nat Phos, Calc Phos, Ferr Phos, Nat
                    Sulph, Nat Mur
                caused by....Calc Phos
                constant....Kali Phos
                epigastrium, in
                two hours after, about....Nat Phos
                worse from eating even small amounts of
                    food....Calc Phos
        general, in....Ferr Phos
        pressure and fullness at the pit of the stomach,
          with....Kali  Sulph
        region of stomach, in....Silica, Mag Phos
        tight band around body, feels like....Mag Phos
pastry disagrees....Kali Mur
pressure
        general sensation in stomach....Mag Phos
        load, as of a....Kali Sulph
        pit of stomach, at....Kali Sulph
        tender to touch in epigastrium....Ferr Phos
pylorus, induration of....Silica
regurgitation (see Vomiting)
risings (see Eructations)
sensations
        fullness, of....Kali Sulph
        nervous empty feeling ....Kali Phos, Nat Phos, Kali
          Sulph
        sickness, deathly....Ferr Phos
        sore, tender to touch....Calc Phos, Ferr Phos
sour breath, and vomit resembles curdled milk....Nat Phos
spasms with griping....Mag Phos
stimulants, intolerance to....Silica

swollen....Ferr Phos
tight clothing around waist is intolerable....Nat Sulph
tongue coatings (see Tongue)
troubles; indigestion, loss of appetite (see also Appetite, Gastric
    Disturbances, Dyspepsia)....Nat Phos, Ferr Phos
ulcerations
        coats surface of stomach to protect....Calc Sulph
        gastric....Nat Phos, Kali Phos, Kali Mur
        general, in....Nat Phos, Kali Phos, Silica
weakness and sinking sensation in....Nat Mur

STOMATITIS (see Mouth)

STONES (see Bladder, Kidney, Gallstones)

STOOL
acid....Nat Phos, Nat Sulph
bilious....Nat Sulph
black; may be thin and offensive smelling....Kali Sulph, Nat
    Sulph
blood, from causes other than hemorrhoids....Calc Sulph, Nat
    Sulph, Kali Phos, Kali Mur, Ferr Phos
brown, dark, bloody, offensive....Kali Phos
cadaverous smelling....Silica
children, when stool is bloody, dry or whitish-yellow....Calc Sulph
clay-colored....Kali Mur, Nat Sulph
coagulated, cheesy-looking....Nat Phos
constant urge to stool....Kali Mur
dark colored
        diarrhea, associated with....Nat Sulph
        general, in....Kali Phos, Nat Sulph
copious....Calc Phos, Ferr Phos
creamy....Nat Phos
crumbling....Nat Mur
diarrhea (see Diarrhea)
dry
        crumbling, and....Nat Mur
        fissures produced in rectum, with....Nat Mur
expelled
        difficulty, with; if soft stool add Nat Sulph....Nat Mur,
            Kali Phos, Silica, Calc Fluor
        extremely hard to move....Kali Phos
        force, with....Mag Phos

inability to....Calc Fluor, Silica

flocculent-resembling shreds or tufts of cotton or containing
    whitish shreds of mucus....Kali Mur
frequent
        general, in....Nat Sulph, Ferr Phos, Nat Phos
        urge, but not able to expel....Calc Phos, Kali Phos, Mag
            Phos
foul, offensive....Kali Phos, Kali Sulph, Silica
frothy....Nat Mur
green
        bilious, and....Nat Sulph
        dark, from excess bile....Silica
        general, in....Nat Sulph, Nat Phos, Calc Phos
hard....Nat Mur, Nat Sulph, Ferr Phos, Calc Phos
hot, sputtering; often noisy and offensive....Calc Phos
ineffectual urging to stool....Kali Sulph
involuntary....Nat Mur
insufficient....Calc Sulph
jelly-like masses....Nat Phos
knotty....Nat Sulph
large mass, very....Nat Sulph
light-colored....Kali Mur
loose (see also Diarrhea)
        elderly, in....Nat Sulph
        jelly-like, and....Nat Phos, Nat Sulph
        morning, in....Nat Mur, Nat Sulph
        watery stools, with....Nat Mur
        worse in cold, wet weather....Nat Sulph
noisy....Calc Phos
offensive....Kali Sulph, Kali Phos, Calc Phos, Silica
painful....Ferr Phos
pale, yellow; associated with diarrhea....Kali Mur
profuse....Calc Phos
purulent....Calc Sulph, Calc Phos
recede when partly expelled....Silica
retain, difficult to....Nat Mur
retention of....Nat Mur
rice water, like....Kali Phos
sacrum pain after stool....Calc Phos
scanty....Nat Phos

slimy....Kali Mur, Kali Sulph, Calc Sulph, Nat Mur, Calc Phos
soreness and tenderness, with....Ferr Phos
sour smelling....Nat Phos
smarting after stool....Nat Mur
sputtering....Calc Phos
straining at....Nat Phos
sudden....Ferr Phos, Nat Phos
tenesmus....Kali Phos
torn feeling after....Nat Mur
undigested food, with....Ferr Phos, Calc Phos
watery
    offensive, noisy....Calc Phos
    soreness, smarting....Nat Mur
white....Kali Mur, Nat Phos, Nat Sulph, Nat Mur
yellow....Kali Sulph, Nat Phos

### STRAINS

first-aid remedy....Ferr Phos
general, in; use topically as a compress....Ferr Phos, Kali Mur, Calc Fluor
muscles; from too much work and a sensation of heat surging through them....Calc Sulph, Mag Phos
pain of....Mag Phos
shock and after-effects of....Nat Sulph
spasm, with....Mag Phos
suppuration, with....Calc Sulph
swelling, with....Ferr Phos, Kali Mur
tendons or ligaments, of (see Sprains)

### STRENGTH (see Muscular Conditions, Vitality)

### STRICTURE....Calc Fluor, Silica, Kali Mur

### STROKE, dissolves the fibrinous exudate that could be pressing on the brain and causing pressure to the affected part....Kali Mur

### STYES

chronic conditions; use 12X potency....Silica
general, in, for pus formation....Silica
inflammation, with....Calc Fluor, Ferr Phos, Silica
internally and/or externally....Silica, Ferr Phos

### STUFFINESS (see Nose)

### ST. VITUS' DANCE-CHOREA, any other remedy may be given

according to symptoms....Calc Phos, Mag Phos, Kali Phos

## SUBLUXATIONS

after treatment....Mag Phos, Kali Mur, Ferr Phos

before manipulation a few tablets of Mag Phos in hot water will relax the muscles and prove an aid to the manipulator....Mag Phos

maintains corrections of manipulations and capsular malalignment; especially useful in joints subjected to stress, such as cervicals, sacro-iliac, knee, shoulder, elbow, wrist, and phalanges....Calc Fluor

## SUNBURN....Nat Mur, Ferr Phos, Kali Sulph, Kali Mur

## SUN HEAT, ill effects of....Ferr Phos

## SUNSTROKE

general, in; give Kali Phos and Kali Sulph, but less frequently; dissolve a few tablets in hot water; take teaspoon full doses every few minutes....Nat Mur

inflammatory symptoms, for; helps respiration....Ferr Phos, Nat Mur

primary remedy to regulate the distribution of moisture; give at frequent intervals....Nat Mur

## SUPPURATION

all cases, for....Silica

bone, of....Calc Fluor, Silica, Calc Sulph

chief remedy....Calc Sulph

dirty, foul....Kali Phos

easily; follow with Calc Sulph....Silica

fever, during suppurative process....Silica

general, in....Calc Sulph, Silica, Nat Phos

glands, of....Silica, Calc Sulph

hard edges, with....Calc Fluor

hastens suppuration and the resolution of suppurative processes; facilitates the reabsorption of exudates; examples are carbuncles, furuncles, abscesses; in any skin condition follow with Calc Sulph....Silica

increases suppuration of wounds and abscesses....Silica

lesions, particularly of surfaces or cavities accessible for drainage where there is a thick, yellowish discharge....Calc Sulph

long continued, such as abscesses and wounds, which do not heal readily and tend to become septic....Calc Sulph

middle ear, if (see also Ears)....Calc Fluor, Ferr Phos
pain, with; can arise from neglected injuries....Silica
promotes; breaks up pathological accumulations....Silica
restrain, to....Calc Sulph
salivary glands, of....Silica
thick, yellow, heavy; can be mixed with blood....Calc Sulph
wounds, of....Calc Sulph, Silica

SURGICAL OPERATIONS
promotes recovery....Ferr Phos, Kali Phos, Calc Phos
before operations give a few doses of....Kali Phos

SWEATING (see Perspiration)

SWELLINGS
blows, cuts and bruises, from....Kali Mur
general, in....Nat Sulph
glandular; chief remedy....Kali Mur
hard swelling anywhere....Calc Fluor
motion brings on pain....Kali Mur
mucous membranes, of....Silica
soft; accompanied by white fibrinous discharge....Kali Mur
uric acid deposits, due to (see also Gout)....Nat Phos

SWALLOWING (see Throat)

SYNOVITIS
acute....Ferr Phos, Calc Fluor, Kali Mur
chronic; a wide bandage may be gently wrung out in a solution of
the salts and bound around the affected area, but not tightly;
renew every three hours....Calc Fluor, Silica
fluid infiltration, helps disperse....Nat Sulph
general, in....Nat Mur
knee, with swelling and difficult movement; chronic....Silica
pain, stiffness and inflammation....Ferr Phos
slow to respond to treatment; chronic....Calc Fluor

SYPHILIS
aggravation, evening....Kali Sulph
caries, syphilitic....Silica
chancre
had in the past....Calc Fluor
phagedenic-sloughing ulcer that spreads....Kali Phos
soft....Kali Mur

chronic....Silica, Kali Mur, Nat Mur, Calc Fluor
condyle, in....Kali Mur
ozena....Nat Sulph
sore throat from....Kali Mur
suppuration stage....Calc Sulph, Silica, Calc Phos
tabes dorsalis
> general, in....Silica, Kali Mur
> paralytic condition of....Silica

SYCOSIS....Nat Sulph

TALKING (see Speech)

TASTE IN MOUTH
acid....Silica, Nat Phos, Nat Mur
acrid....Calc Sulph
bad
> general, in....Nat Sulph, Kali Phos
> morning, in....Calc Phos

bitter
> general, in—-Nat Sulph, Kali Mur, Kali Phos
> morning, in....Calc Phos, Calc Fluor

coppery....Nat Phos
disgusting....Calc Phos
insipid....Kali Sulph, Calc Sulph
loss of....Nat Mur, Kali Sulph
regain, to, with yellow discharge....Kali Sulph
salty....Nat Mur
soapy....Calc Sulph
sour....Nat Mur, Calc Sulph, Nat Phos

TEETH
abscess at the roots (see also Abscess)....Silica
ache
> alternates with frontal headache....Kali Phos
> aggravates
>> cold things....Mag Phos
>> food....Calc Fluor
>> warmth....Kali Sulph
> bed, after going to....Mag Phos
> changes places rapidly....Mag Phos
> chilling of feet causes....Silica
> congestive....Ferr Phos, Mag Phos

dental fistula, with....Silica
excessive flow of saliva or tears, with....Nat Mur
feverish, and....Nat Mur, Mag Phos
gums bleeding easily, with....Kali Phos
hot cheek, with....Ferr Phos
inflammation, soreness; if swelling give Kali Mur....Ferr
   Phos, Mag Phos
neuralgic (see also Neuralgia)....Mag Phos, Nat Mur
pain (see also Pain)
        boring....Calc Phos
        deep-seated....Silica
        intense rheumatic toothache....Mag Phos
        shooting, spasmodic, shifting....Mag Phos
        tingling....Calc Phos
relieves
        cold air....Kali Sulph, Nat Sulph
        cool air....Kali Sulph
        hot liquids....Mag Phos
        smoking of tobacco....Nat Sulph
        water....Ferr Phos, Nat Sulph
rheumatic....Calc Sulph
salivation, with....Nat Mur
swelling
        gums and cheeks, of....Calc Sulph
        hard on cheeks, with toothache....Calc Fluor
swollen cheek, with....Kali Mur, Calc Sulph
tears, involuntary flow of....Nat Mur
ulceration, with (see Ulcerations)....Silica, Calc Sulph
warm food, after....Ferr Phos
worse
        evening, in....Kali Sulph
        night, at....Silica, Calc Phos
backwardness, with bone weakness or recurring tooth
   troubles....Calc Fluor
bleeding after extractions; with swelling alternate with Kali
   Mur....Ferr Phos
bone ailments....Calc Fluor
chattering, nervous....Kali Phos
clenched....Mag Phos
decay
        pain, with....Kali Phos

rapidly; also treat as for enamel deficiency....Calc Phos,
Calc Fluor

deposits on teeth, brown....Kali Phos

develops slowly....Calc Phos

drooling....Nat Mur

enamel

brittle....Calc Fluor

defective....Calc Fluor

deficiencies....Calc Fluor, Calc Phos, Silica

harden, helps to....Mag Phos

rough and thin....Calc Fluor, Calc Phos

fistula....Silica

formation of, aids....Calc Phos

grinding

during sleep....Nat Phos, Kali Phos

general, in....Nat Phos, Kali Phos

grits teeth....Nat Phos

gums (see  Gums)

loose

general, in....Calc Fluor, Silica, Nat Mur, Calc Phos

sockets, in their, and decay rapidly; there may be pain;
alternate with Calc Phos....Calc Fluor

long, too....Ferr Phos

malnutrition of teeth....Calc Fluor

neuralgia, with (see also Neuralgia)....Mag Phos, Nat Mur

pain

dentistry, associated with....Nat Sulph

general, in....Mag Phos

inflammation and soreness, with....Ferr Phos

severe

filled or decayed teeth, in....Kali Phos

shooting....Ferr Phos

pregnancy, ailments of teeth during....Calc Phos, Calc Fluor

primary remedy for the teeth; Silica is also an important
remedy....Calc Fluor

saliva, excessive, with....Nat Mur

sensitive

cold air or touch, to....Mag Phos

general, in; also dissolve in water and applied externally
with a cotton swab....Calc Fluor, Calc Sulph, Mag

Phos, Kali Phos
slow development and rapid decay....Calc Fluor
soreness....Kali Phos, Ferr Phos
ulcerations, with (see also Ulcerations)....Calc Sulph, Silica
worse touch, cold air, cold water; cannot brush with cold
water....Mag Phos

TEETHING
complaints of children during teething
general, in....Calc Phos
spasmodic symptoms, especially....Mag Phos
convulsions, with....Mag Phos, Calc Phos, Ferr Phos
coughs
dry, spasmodic, with twitching....Mag Phos
during teething....Calc Phos
cramps, with....Mag Phos
crying of infants during teething period; will prevent many
unpleasant, restless, and crying spells....Calc Phos
delayed....Calc Fluor, Silica
diarrhea, with....Nat Phos
difficult....Calc Phos, Silica
drooling of saliva by infant....Nat Mur
feverish....Ferr Phos, Kali Sulph
gastric problem, with....Nat Phos
general, in....Nat Phos, Calc Phos, Calc Fluor
gums swollen; no teeth yet fretful and feverish; give every 2 hours
if acute....Ferr Phos, Calc Phos
marasmus, with....Calc Phos
pain, with; dissolve remedy in hot water for better effects; if
symptoms are better with cold applications give Ferr Phos
instead....Mag Phos
pale face when teething is difficult....Calc Phos
poor nutrition and slow development, related to....Calc Phos
problems with; chief remedy....Calc Phos
retarded development....Calc Phos
slow....Calc Phos, Silica
stools increased, with....Nat Mur
summer complaints in teething children....Calc Phos

TELANGIECTASIS, spider web dilations of surface veins....Ferr Phos,
Calc Fluor

TEMPERATURE (see Fever)

TENDONS

cracking of....Kali Mur, Ferr Phos
inflammation of a tendon sheath with a crackling sound-Tenalgia
      crepitans....Ferr Phos, Calc Fluor, Kali Mur, Nat Phos
sprained (see Sprains)....Ferr Phos, Mag Phos

TESTICLES (see Sexual Organs, Male)

THIGH (see also Extremities)

drawing sensation inside thigh....Nat Phos
soreness....Calc Phos

THIRST

burning....Kali Sulph, Calc Sulph, Nat Mur
dry mouth, with....Calc Phos
evening, during....Nat Sulph
excessive....Nat Mur
extreme....Nat Mur
general, in....Ferr Phos
increased, with fever....Nat Mur
sugary drinks, for....Mag Phos
thirstless

      general, in....Kali Phos
      worse with hot drinks....Kali Sulph
violent....Nat Mur
water or drinks, cold, for....Ferr Phos, Kali Phos, Mag Phos

THROAT

burning

      pharynx; cases of chronic catarrh where there is excessive
            mucus from the posterior nares....Calc Phos
      red throat, with....Ferr Phos, Calc Phos
choking....Mag Phos
colds (see Colds)
congestion of throat, spasmodic....Mag Phos, Ferr Phos
constriction; along with chest constriction....Mag Phos, Nat Mur
deglutition-act of swallowing
      painful....Ferr Phos, Calc Phos, Kali Mur
      swallow, must....Mag Phos
diphtheria (see Diphtheria)
diphtheritic sore....Kali Mur
dryness of....Nat Mur, Ferr Phos, Nat Sulph, Nat Phos, Kali Phos
enlargement of....Nat Mur

epiglottis feels closed....Calc Fluor
expectoration (see Expectoration)
exudation (see Exudation)
fauces-the cavity of the throat
        inflamed....Ferr Phos
        painful....Ferr Phos
        red....Ferr Phos
        swollen....Calc Sulph
gangrenous....Kali Phos
glands (see Glands)
glottis, spasm of....Calc Phos, Mag Phos
goiter (see Goiter)
grayish patches in....Kali Mur
heat in throat....Ferr Phos
heat, pain and dryness, with; give frequently during the acute
   stage until inflammation subsides....Ferr Phos
hoarseness (see Hoarseness)
inflamed (see also Inflammation)
        general, in....Ferr Phos, Nat Sulph, Nat Phos
        mucous membrane lining; watery secretion....Nat Mur
        swelling, with, and grayish-white patches....Kali Mur
larynx (see Larynx)
lump in, on swallowing....Nat Sulph, Nat Phos, Nat Mur
malignant conditions in....Kali Phos
membranous exudations in throat (see also Diphtheria)....Kali
   Mur
mucus (see also Expectoration)
        fills the mouth in the morning, with difficulty
           swallowing; hoarseness that is worse evening; tough
           mucus....Kali Sulph
        salty, raised from throat....Kali Phos, Nat Phos
        throat covered with transparent mucus....Nat Mur
        tough....Kali Sulph
palate (see Palate)
pain (see also Pain)
        general, in....Calc Phos, Ferr Phos
        pharynx (see Pharynx)
        redness, but no exudation....Ferr Phos
        sticking-type pain on swallowing....Calc Phos
        swallowing, on....Kali Mur, Mag Phos

posterior nares
> burning sensation in pharynx; chronic catarrh,
> > excessive....Calc Phos
> mucus drops from....Nat Phos

quinsy (see Quinsy)

red, dry, inflamed, painful....Ferr Phos

relaxed
> general, in....Calc Fluor
> relaxed uvula, with, causing irritation, tickling and
> > cough....Calc Fluor, Calc Phos, Nat Mur

scraping feeling when talking....Calc Phos

sensations
> ball rising in throat, like a....Kali Phos
> choking in throat....Mag Phos
> lump in throat when swallowing....Nat Sulph, Nat Phos,
> > Nat Mur
> plug has lodged in throat, as if....Nat Mur
> suffocative feeling in throat....Mag Phos

sore
> acute stage, until inflammation subsides....Ferr Phos
> ache, and, with pain on swallowing....Calc Phos
> catarrhal (see Discharge, Expectoration, Catarrh)
> chief remedies; sip frequently after dissolving 6 tablets of
> > each remedy in one cup water; take as needed....Ferr
> > Phos, Kali Mur
> chronic
> > deafness, with....Kali Mur
> > general, in....Nat Mur
> clergyman's sore throat....Calc Phos, Ferr Phos
> dryness, excessive, or too much secretion....Nat Mur
> first sign of, especially with redness and swelling....Calc Sulph
> first stage with pain, heat, redness....Ferr Phos, Calc Sulph
> gangrenous....Kali Phos
> general, in....Nat Mur, Ferr Phos, Kali Mur, Calc Fluor,
> > Kali Phos
> pain, with
> > burning, red throat; dry; hoarseness, loss of
> > > voice....Ferr Phos
> > much pain....Ferr Phos
> > stinging when swallowing; neck being painful
> > > to touch....Silica

stitching....Nat Mur
swallowing, on....Calc Phos, Mag Phos
throbbing....Ferr Phos
raw feeling, with; throat inflamed with creamy, yellow,
    moist coating; also inflamed tonsils....Nat Phos
relaxed; add to hot water or take after meals....Calc
    Phos, Calc Fluor
singing or public speaking, from....Ferr Phos, Calc Phos
stiff, and....Mag Phos
syphilitic sore throat....Kali Mur
spasm....Mag Phos
suppuration of....Calc Sulph, Silica
swallow
    choking on attempting to....Mag Phos
    constant desire to....Kali Phos
    dysphagia
        general, in....Nat Mur, Kali Mur
        obstruction in throat; take remedies in a small
            amount of hot water, with frequent
            sips....Silica, Mag Phos
    liquids give sensation of constriction....Mag Phos
    lump in throat when swallowing....Nat Sulph, Nat Phos,
    Nat Mur
    must....Mag Phos
    painful....Calc Phos, Kali Mur, Ferr Phos
    sticking pain, with....Calc Phos
    stinging pain, with, and neck painful to touch....Silica
swollen (see also Swellings, Glands, Tonsils)
    glands and tonsils, of....Kali Mur, Ferr Phos
    inflamed with grayish-white patches....Kali Mur
symptoms with dry, painful nose....Nat Mur
thrush (see Thrush)
tickling
    enlarged soft palate, from....Calc Fluor
    general, in....Calc Fluor
    larynx, in....Calc Sulph, Calc Phos
tightness in throat, with excess mucus and a pressing pain
    when swallowing....Calc Sulph
tonsils (see Tonsils)
ulcerated (see also Ulcerations)
    fever and pain, with....Ferr Phos

general, in....Kali Mur, Nat Phos, Ferr Phos, Nat Sulph,
Nat Mur

thick, yellow discharge....Silica

white or gray patches....Kali Mur

uvula

causing cough....Calc Fluor

elongated....Nat Mur

inflamed....Nat Mur, Ferr Phos

relaxed, causing irritation, tickling and cough....Nat
Mur, Calc Fluor, Calc Phos

vocal cords (see Voice)

windpipe, spasmodic closure of....Mag Phos

THROMBOSIS, formation of a blood clot....Ferr Phos, Kali Mur, Calc Fluor

THRUSH

children, in....Kali Mur

general....Kali Mur, Nat Mur

saliva excessive, with....Nat Mur

THUMBS (see Hands, Fingers)

THYROID GLAND (see Glands)

TINEA (see Fungus)

TINNITUS (see Ear, noises)

TIRED FEELING (see Vitality, Fatigue)

TISSUE

cleans out accumulated non-functional organic matter, and causes
infiltrated parts to discharge their contents readily, throwing
off decaying organic matter so not to cause injury to the
surrounding tissues....Calc Sulph

exudates (see Exudates)

fibers, elastic, relaxed....Calc Fluor

nervous tissue; nutritional and functional remedy (see also
Nutritional, Nerves)....Mag Phos

scaly, becomes....Kali Sulph, Calc Phos, Nat Mur, Kali Mur

septic conditions (see also Cleanser)....Kali Phos, Silica

swelling, from blows, cuts and bruises....Kali Mur

tone, restores, to tissues and weakened organs....Calc Phos

unhealthy....Calc Sulph

water-logged....Nat Sulph

TOES (see Feet)

TONGUE

blisters on tip of....Nat Mur, Nat Sulph, Nat Phos, Calc Phos
clean
> dry, and; sometimes Ferr Phos is also useful....Mag Phos,
> Nat Mur
> general, in....Ferr Phos, Nat Mur, Mag Phos
> inflammatory condition, with....Ferr Phos
> moist....Nat Phos

cleaves to roof of mouth, or feels as if it will....Kali Phos
coating on tongue
> brown
>> dark....Kali Phos, Nat Sulph
>> dirty, with vomiting of bile....Nat Sulph
> brownish
>> brownish-green....Nat Sulph
>> brownish-yellow, or yellow coating....Nat Sulph
>> general, in....Kali Phos, Nat Sulph
> clean....Ferr Phos
> clear; may be accompanied by slimy, watery, frothy,
> transparent coating....Nat Mur
> clay-colored....Calc Sulph
> creamy or creamy golden-yellow....Nat Phos
> dirty greenish-gray or brown on root of tongue with
> saliva....Nat Sulph
> fur....Kali Mur, Ferr Phos
> golden-yellow, or with golden-yellow creamy coating at
> the root of the tongue; whole tongue sometimes
> appears like wash leather....Nat Phos
> grayish
>> general, in....Kali Mur, Nat Sulph
>> grayish-green....Nat Sulph
>> grayish-white....Kali Mur
> green....Nat Sulph
> greenish-gray....Nat Sulph
> moist, creamy, on back part....Nat Phos
> mustard-looking, brownish, stale; breath offensive....Kali
> Phos
> slimy....Kali Mur
> white

edges, on....Kali Sulph
fur....Calc Phos, Kali Mur
general, in....Kali Mur, Kali Sulph, Calc Phos
gray-white or with excessive fibrinous secretions;
    may be associated with diarrhea....Kali Mur
yellow
    base, at....Calc Sulph
    bright fur....Nat Phos
    general, in....Kali Sulph, Nat Phos
    slimy, and....Kali Sulph
cracked....Calc Fluor
dirty looking....Nat Sulph
    general, in....Kali Sulph, Nat Sulph, Kali Phos
    greenish-gray or greenish-brown....Nat Sulph
dry
    excessive in morning....Kali Phos, Nat Mur, Kali Mur
    low fevers, in; watery discharge from bowels....Nat Mur
    morning, in....Kali Phos
edges
    froth-covered....Nat Mur
    red and sore....Kali Phos
    white....Kali Sulph
flabby....Calc Sulph
frothy....Nat Mur
hair, sensation of, on the tongue; general, in....Silica, Nat Mur
hair, sensation of, on tip....Nat Phos
hardening, after inflammation....Calc Fluor
induration of....Calc Fluor, Silica
inflammation
    dryness, with....Kali Phos
    exhaustion, with....Kali Phos
    general, in....Ferr Phos, Nat Phos, Nat Sulph, Mag Phos
    suppuration, with....Calc Sulph, Silica
    swelling, with....Kali Mur, Ferr Phos
mapped....Nat Mur, Kali Mur, Nat Sulph, Calc Fluor
moist....Nat Phos, Nat Mur
numb....Calc Phos, Nat Mur
pimples on....Calc Phos
ranula-large cystic tumor....Nat Mur
red
    bright, with rawness....Mag Phos

dark, with swelling or inflammation....Ferr Phos
general, in....Ferr Phos, Nat Sulph, Mag Phos, Nat Phos
rheumatic conditions, associated with yellow tongue and other
acid symptoms involving the mouth and sweat glands....Nat
Phos
saliva bubbles on tongue....Nat Mur
scalded, as if....Mag Phos
sensation as if tongue would cleave to roof of mouth....Kali Phos
slimy....Kali Sulph, Kali Phos, Nat Mur, Nat Sulph, Kali Mur
stiff....Calc Phos, Nat Mur
swelling
    chronic....Calc Fluor
    dark red....Ferr Phos
    general, in....Kali Mur, Calc Phos
taste (see Taste)
ulceration....Silica
vesicles on....Nat Mur

## TONIC

beauty....Ferr Phos, Kali Phos
constitutional; after prolonged nursing, leukorrhea, etc....Calc
Phos

## TONSILS

abscess (see also Abscess)....Calc Sulph, Silica
chronic enlargement; may cause pain when open mouth;
difficulty swallowing....Calc Phos
creamy, yellow, moist coating on....Nat Phos
discoloration, spots....Kali Mur
enlarged
    chronic....Calc Phos
    deafness, with....Calc Phos
    general, in....Calc Fluor, Calc Phos, Kali Phos, Nat Mur
    inflamed....Kali Phos, Ferr Phos
    periodically....Silica
eruptions, pustules (see also Eruptions, Pustules)....Kali Mur
exudate (see Exudate)
gray-white patches on....Kali Mur
inflammation of or Tonsillitis
    acute....Ferr Phos
    chronic; precede with Ferr Phos in the primary or acute
    stage....Kali Mur

creamy, yellow, moist coating, with; throat also
inflamed....Nat Phos

deafness, with, and much swelling....Kali Mur, Calc
Phos

discharge of matter; if an abscess forms (see also
Discharge, Abscess, Pus).,.,Calc Sulph

general, in; give Silica when pus begins to form....Ferr
Phos, Kali Mur, Calc Fluor, Nat Phos

last stage when discharge is purulent....Calc Sulph

pain on opening mouth....Calc Phos

red, painful when swallowing....Ferr Phos

suppuration (see also Suppuration)....Silica, Calc Sulph

swelling, with....Kali Mur

indurated....Calc Fluor

large, indurated, relaxed throat and uvula elongated....Calc Fluor

pain of; accompanied by soft swellings....Kali Mur

primary remedy....Ferr Phos

quinsy (see Quinsy)

secondary remedy; when swelling starts....Kali Mur

sore....Kali Phos

spots, white or gray....Kali Mur

suppuration threatening....Silica

swelling, with sore throat....Kali Mur, Ferr Phos

swollen, red and enlarged....Calc Phos

white deposit on....Kali Phos

yellow coating on....Nat Phos

TOOTHACHE (see Teeth, ache)

TOXIC, THE ANTI-TOXIC CELL SALTS (see also Cleanser)....Kali
Sulph, Nat Mur

TRAUMA (see Blows, Nervous States, Accidents, Injuries, First-Aid)

TREMORS (see also Muscular, Nerves)....Mag Phos

TUBERCULOSIS

constitutional; with night sweats....Silica, Calc Sulph

general, in....Calc Sulph, Nat Phos, Silica, Calc Phos

swelling of glands, with....Nat Phos, Kali Mur

TUMORS

bloody....Calc Fluor

breast, of....Calc Fluor

encysted....Calc Fluor, Calc Sulph
eyelids, of...Calc Fluor
osseous....Calc Fluor
scalp, on....Calc Fluor
vascular....Calc Fluor

## TWITCHING (see Muscular, Nerves)

## ULCERATED STOMACH (see Stomach, ulcerations)

## ULCERATIONS

all types....Silica
bone, of....Silica, Calc Fluor, Calc Sulph
extremities, of....Kali Mur
fistulous
>    feet, about....Calc Phos
>    general, in....Silica, Calc Fluor
>    thick, yellow pus, with....Silica, Calc Fluor, Calc Sulph
general, in (also treat as for Abscess)....Silica, Calc Sulph
indolent....Calc Phos, Silica, Calc Fluor
inflamed....Ferr Phos
intestinal....Calc Sulph
mouth, of (see Mouth, ulcers)
mucous membranes and skin, of....Calc Sulph
nails, around....Silica
proud flesh, with....Silica, Kali Mur, Calc Sulph
purulent....Silica, Calc Sulph
scrofulous....Calc Phos
skin oozing....Calc Sulph
stomach (see Stomach, ulcerations)
syphilitic (see also Syphilis)....Silica, Calc Phos, Calc Sulph
varicose....Calc Fluor

## UNSTEADY HANDWRITING (see Muscular, Nerves)

## URETHRA

bleeding from....Kali Phos
cutting pains after urination....Nat Mur, Calc Phos, Kali Phos
itching in....Kali Phos
pain in urethra and neck of bladder....Calc Phos
sore to pressure....Nat Mur

## URIC ACID DEPOSITS (see Gout)

URINE (see also Bladder Disorders)

    albuminous....Kali Sulph, Kali Mur, Calc Phos, Kali Phos

    bile, loaded with....Nat Sulph

    blood in urine

        general, in....Ferr Phos, Nat Mur, Kali Phos

        scurvy, from....Nat Mur

    burning

        after urination....Nat Mur, Ferr Phos

        during urination....Nat Sulph

        pain over kidneys....Ferr Phos

    calculous phosphates in....Calc Phos

    colored urine, highly

        general, in....Ferr Phos, Calc Phos

        fever, with....Ferr Phos, Nat Phos

    copious....Nat Mur, Calc Fluor, Calc Phos

    dark colored urine with sandy deposits; may be accompanied
      with rheumatism....Kali Mur, Nat Phos, Nat Sulph

    deposits

        brick dust sediment....Silica, Nat Sulph

        clings to side of vessels....Nat Sulph

        flocculent sediment in....Calc Phos

        gravel (see Urine, gravel)

        lithic....Nat Sulph

        sandy and dark colored urine....Kali Mur, Nat Phos, Nat
          Sulph

    enuresis (see Enuresis)

    excessive flow

        general, in....Ferr Phos, Nat Sulph, Nat Phos

        polyuria simplex....Mag Phos, Calc Phos, Ferr Phos, Nat
          Phos, Nat Mur, Nat Sulph

        watery urine, of....Nat Mur, Ferr Phos

    frequency

        elderly, in....Kali Phos

        general, in....Ferr Phos, Nat Mur

        inability to retain urine, and with acidity....Nat Phos,
          Ferr Phos

        urge, and....Mag Phos, Ferr Phos, Nat Phos, Calc Phos,
          Nat Sulph

        water-like, excess, sometimes scalding....Kali Phos

gravel
        bilious persons, in....Nat Sulph
        general, in....Silica, Calc Phos, Mag Phos, Nat Sulph
        gouty symptoms, with....Nat Sulph
        pain while passing....Mag Phos, Nat Sulph
        sediment in urine....Calc Phos, Nat Sulph
incontinence (see Enuresis, Bed Wetting)
increased urine....Calc Phos, Nat Sulph, Ferr Phos, Nat Mur
intermittent flow....Nat Phos
mucus and pus, loaded with....Silica, Nat Sulph
odor, pungent....Calc Fluor
phosphates in....Calc Phos
pus and mucus, loaded with....Nat Sulph, Silica
red and hectic....Calc Sulph
retention of urine
        general, in....Mag Phos
        spasmodic....Nat Phos, Mag Phos
scanty....Calc Fluor
scalding....Kali Phos
sugar in....Nat Sulph
suppression, urinary....Ferr Phos
urates in....Silica, Calc Sulph
urge is frequent....Mag Phos, Ferr Phos, Nat Phos, Calc Phos, Nat Sulph
uric acid, excess of (see also Gout)....Silica, Kali Mur
watery, excessive flow, with great thirst....Nat Mur, Ferr Phos
yellow-like saffron....Kali Phos
yellowish-green....Nat Sulph

URTICARIA (see Hives)

UTERINE DISPLACEMENT (see Uterus)

UTERUS
aching in....Calc Phos
burning in....Nat Mur
congestion, chronic....Kali Mur, Calc Fluor
cutting pain in....Nat Mur
displacements; with rheumatic or dragging pains....Calc Phos, Calc Fluor
hypertrophy of....Kali Mur
inflammation of....Kali Mur
muscle tone loose after miscarriage....Calc Fluor

prolapse
>> sinking feeling, with....Nat Phos, Calc Phos
>> sitting relieves....Nat Mur
>> womb, with dragging pains....Calc Fluor
> ulceration (see also Ulcerations)....Kali Mur, Silica
> weakness and distress in....Nat Phos, Calc Phos

## UVULA (see Throat)

## VACCINATION, after effects of....Kali Mur, Ferr Phos, Nat Phos, Nat Mur, Silica

## VAGINAL

cysts, serous....Silica
discharge (see also Leukorrhea, Exudations)
>> acid....Nat Phos
>> creamy....Nat Phos, Calc Phos
>> creamy, especially when flow is thick or comes in gushes....Silica
>> deep red or blackish-red....Kali Phos
>> general, in....Kali Mur, Calc Phos
>> irritation, with....Kali Mur
>> scalding, smarting....Nat Mur, Kali Phos
>> sickening....Nat Phos
>> slimy, yellow or greenish....Kali Sulph
>> sour smelling....Nat Phos
>> thick
>>> offensive odor, with....Kali Phos
>>> white, bland....Kali Mur
>> watery, creamy yellow....Nat Phos, Nat Mur, Kali Sulph
>> white....Kali Mur
>> yellow....Kali Sulph, Kali Phos
dryness
>> excessive....Nat Mur, Ferr Phos
>> hot, and....Ferr Phos
herpes (see Herpes)
inflammation (see Inflammation)
itching (see also Itching)
>> general, in....Calc Phos, Kali Phos, Nat Phos
>> severe....Kali Phos
pain, burning and soreness, after urination....Nat Mur, Ferr Phos
sensitive....Silica, Ferr Phos
spasms, constrictive....Mag Phos

vaginismus-painful spasms of vagina....Ferr Phos, Mag Phos

VARICOCELE....Ferr Phos, Calc Fluor, Silica

VEINS (see also Blood Vessels)

> spider web dilations of surface veins....Ferr Phos, Calc Fluor
> varicose veins
>> enlarged; all varicose veins....Calc Fluor, Silica, Nat Mur, Ferr Phos
>> general, in....Ferr Phos, Calc Fluor, Silica, Nat Mur
>> primary remedies....Calc Fluor, Silica
>> ulcerations (see also Ulcerations)....Calc Fluor
>> young people, in....Ferr Phos

VERTIGO

> acid producing gastric problems, accompanied by....Nat Phos
> anemia, with....Kali Phos
> cold feeling in head, with....Calc Phos
> dizziness, with (see also Dizziness)....Kali Phos
> elderly, in....Calc Phos
> fall to the left side, tendency to....Silica
> gastric derangements, from....Nat Sulph, Nat Phos
> general, in....Calc Phos, Silica, Ferr Phos, Kali Phos, Nat Sulph
> giddiness
>> blood rushing to the head, from, with flushing, throbbing or pressing pain....Ferr Phos
>> bitter taste in the mouth, with; inclined to fall on the right side with gastric derangement; tongue dirty greenish or green-brown coating at the back....Nat Sulph
>> exhaustion, from, and weakness....Kali Phos
>> swimming of the head, from nervous causes; worse on rising or looking upwards....Kali Phos
> labyrinthitis, from....Silica
> looking upward, from
>> general, in....Kali Phos, Kali Sulph
>> feels like you are falling....Kali Sulph
> motion, on, and when walking....Calc Phos
> nausea, with
>> general, in....Calc Sulph
>> extreme nausea....Calc Phos
> nervous exhaustion, from....Kali Phos
> optical defects, from (see Vision)

rising up, when....Kali Phos, Kali Sulph
rush of blood to the head, from....Ferr Phos
throbbing pain, with, and rush of blood to head....Ferr Phos

**VESICLES** (see also Eruptions)
colorless, watery....Nat Mur
general, in....Calc Phos, Nat Sulph
small, hard, resulted from severe cases of poison ivy that forms
    scabs; apply topically with a cotton swab by dissolving remedy
    in water....Kali Sulph
thick, white contents....Kali Mur
watery....Nat Mur
yellowish water, with....Nat Sulph

**VISION**
blurred
    general, in....Kali Phos, Calc Fluor
    letters run together when reading....Nat Mur
    straining eyes, after....Calc Fluor
color vision abnormal....Mag Phos
colors seen before eyes
    dark....Kali Sulph
    general, in....Mag Phos
double....Nat Mur, Mag Phos, Kali Phos, Calc Sulph
flickering before eyes....Calc Fluor
halo effects....Kali Phos
impaired....Nat Mur
one-half of an object seen, with spasmodic contractions of blood
    vessels serving the retina....Mag Phos
partial....Mag Phos
spots before eyes
    black....Kali Phos, Silica
    dark....-Mag Phos, Kali Mur
    floaters....Silica, Kali Phos
    general, in....Mag Phos
weak
    coitus, after....Kali Phos
    exhaustion, from....Kali Phos

**VITALITY**
debility (see Debility)
failure of strength....Kali Phos
fatigue (see Fatigue)

flagging; acts as a stabilizing influence in the face of
adversity....Kali Phos

general loss of vitality, with....Calc Phos, Mag Phos, Ferr Phos,
Kali Phos

increase, to; also improve diet and increase exercise....Kali Mur

nutrition, all-around, important in....Calc Phos

physical exertion tires you easily....Ferr Phos

regain energy, to; good to take before exercise....Kali Phos, Ferr
Phos

run down feeling; primary remedy....Calc Phos

tired feeling....Ferr Phos, Nat Sulph, Nat Phos, Mag Phos, Nat
Mur, Kali Phos

weak or anemic; increases nutritional tone....Ferr Phos, Calc Phos

## VOICE

hoarseness (see Hoarseness)

huskiness after singing or speaking....Ferr Phos

loss of

cold, from....Ferr Phos, Kali Mur

excessive speaking, from; dissolve in hot water and take
in sips; repeat as needed....Ferr Phos, Kali Mur

general, in....Ferr Phos, Kali Mur, Kali Phos

nervous causes, from....Kali Phos, Mag Phos

paralysis of vocal cords, from....Kali Phos

shrills, suddenly....Mag Phos, Kali Phos

vocal cord straining, from....Kali Phos, Ferr Phos

paralysis of vocal cords....Kali Phos

shrill, coming on suddenly while speaking....Kali Phos, Mag Phos

speaking is causing fatigue....Kali Sulph

## VOMITING

acid vomit....Nat Phos, Nat Sulph, Nat Mur

all conditions when excess of saliva and watery vomiting is
present; tongue has a clear, frothy, transparent coating....Nat
Mur

bile....Nat Sulph

bitter

fluids....Nat Sulph

foods....Kali Phos

blood

bright red....Ferr Phos

clotted blood....Kali Mur

dark blood

     clotted....Ferr Phos, Kali Mur

     general, in....Kali Mur

  food, and....Ferr Phos

  general, in; dissolve a few tablets of each in tepid water
     and sip in an emergency....Ferr Phos, Nat Mur, Kali
     Mur, Calc Fluor, Kali Phos

     viscid....Kali Mur

coffee grounds, like....Kali Phos, Nat Phos, Nat Mur

cold water or drinks, after....Calc Phos

curdled masses....Nat Phos, Nat Mur

fluid, sour....Nat Phos

food

     after eating....Mag Phos

     blood, and....Ferr Phos

     general, in....Ferr Phos

frothy....Nat Mur

general, in; dissolve in warm water and take in sips....Ferr Phos,
  Nat Mur, Kali Mur, Calc Fluor

green, bilious....Nat Sulph, Nat Phos

greenish water....Kali Phos, Nat Sulph

hysterical....Kali Phos, Mag Phos, Nat Mur

ice cream, after....Calc Phos

infants (see also Infant's Problems)

     Mother's milk, of; accompanied with diarrhea; give to
       both mother and baby....Silica

     general, in....Calc Phos

     nursing, immediately after....Silica, Calc Phos, Ferr Phos

     sour, curled milk....Calc Phos, Nat Phos

morning

     breakfast, before....Silica, Ferr Phos

     early, after awakening; chronic condition....Calc Phos

     general, in....Silica

morning sickness (see Morning Sickness)

mucus

     stringy....Nat Mur

     thick, white....Kali Mur

     transparent....Nat Mur, Ferr Phos

     watery....Nat Mur

     white....Kali Mur

nausea, with....Mag Phos

regurgitation of food after eating....Mag Phos
retching....Mag Phos
salty, greenish water....Nat Sulph
sour
        acid fluids, and, during fever....Nat Phos
        fluids, during fever....Nat Phos
        food and blood....Kali Phos
        froth....Nat Phos
        general, in....Ferr Phos, Kali Phos, Nat Mur, Nat Sulph
        smelling....Nat Phos
stomach ache, from....Mag Phos
thick, white phlegm....Kali Mur
transparent slime....Nat Mur
undigested food
        constantly....Calc Fluor
        general, in....Ferr Phos, Nat Phos, Calc Phos, Calc Fluor
        tongue is clean, but....Ferr Phos
watery, looks....Nat Mur

## VULVA (see Sexual Organs, Female)

## WALKING

gait unsteady....Nat Phos
slow in learning....Calc Phos

## WARTS

anus, wart-like eruptions on....Nat Sulph
general, in; a solution of the salts may also be applied externally
    and kept on all night....Kali Mur, Nat Sulph, Silica, Nat Mur
painful....Kali Sulph
palms of hands that are sore to touch, on....Nat Mur, Kali Mur
    Nat Sulph

## WASTING DISEASE (see also Atrophy, Debility)....Kali Phos, Calc Phos

## WATER BALANCE distributing tissue salt; any disorder associated with
a disturbed water balance; examples are a dry mouth, diarrhea, or
an excessive watery discharge; any part of the body that is too
dry or too wet....Nat Mur

## WATER BRASH....Nat Mur, Nat Phos, Kali Phos

## WEAKNESS (see also Vitality, Fatigue, Muscular, Nerves, Debility)

## WHEALS (see also Hives)....Nat Sulph, Nat Mur

WHOOPING COUGH (see Cough)

WHITLOW (see Felon)

WINDPIPE (see Throat)

WOMEN'S PROBLEMS (see Female Disorders)

WORMS
>general, in....Mag Phos, Calc Phos, Nat Phos
>intestinal....Nat Phos, Calc Phos, Ferr Phos
>long type....Nat Phos
>sleep is restless from....Ferr Phos, Nat Phos
>squinting, with....Nat Phos
>stomach ache, with....Nat Phos
>thread-like....Ferr Phos, Nat Phos, Kali Mur

WORSE, SYMPTOMS BECOME
>afternoon....Nat Phos
>alone, when....Kali Sulph, Kali Phos
>cold weather, from....Calc Phos
>damp weather, from....Calc Phos
>evening....Kali Sulph, Nat Phos, Kali Phos
>every other day....Nat Mur
>fresh air....Calc Phos
>morning
>>evening, and; symptoms persist during night....Kali Phos
>>general, in—Nat Mur, Nat Sulph
>night....Silica, Calc Phos
>right-sided....Mag Phos
>ten to eleven a.m.....Nat Mur

WOUNDS, MINOR
>bleeding; apply externally also to the injured parts....Ferr Phos
>cuts, bruises; primary remedy; apply powdered tablets externally whenever possible to alleviate pain (see also Cuts, Bruises)....Ferr Phos
>cleanser of tissues (see Cleanser)
>fresh....Ferr Phos, Kali Phos
>festering, with; thick, yellow pus discharge....Silica
>first-aid (see First Aid)
>heals readily, does not....Calc Sulph
>neglected; there is discharge, pus....Calc Sulph
>pus is white....Silica

septic; give every 2 hours (see also Cleanser)....Kali Phos

shock and after-effects of....Nat Sulph, Nat Mur, Kali Phos

slow to heal....Calc Sulph

suppuration, with (see also Suppuration)....Calc Sulph, Silica

swelling, with....Kali Mur, Ferr Phos

unconscious, if; moisten lips with the indicated remedies....Ferr Phos, Kali Phos

**WRIST**

ache....Nat Phos, Ferr Phos, Calc Phos

pain....Nat Phos

**YAWNING**

a lot; symptoms disappear when things start becoming more interesting or when eating....Kali Phos

constant stretching, and....Calc Phos, Kali Phos

hysterical....Kali Phos

spasmodic....Calc Phos, Mag Phos

# CELL SALT CASE STUDIES

## Case 1

A 31-year-old femald presents with the following symptoms:

• She has muscular spasms and pain, especially in the arms, hands, and feet.
• There is constant tension to the scalp, jaw, and shoulders.
• The symptoms are worse as the day goes on.
• She is worse tightening her fist.
• Her symptoms become worse with emotional stress and movement.
• She has foot cramps often.
• Her extremities are always cold.
• The pain feels dull and vice-like with a pulling sensation.

<u>The correct cell salts are:</u>
MAG PHOS: pain, anti-spasmodic, cramping
NAT SULPH: removes toxic waste from the cells
CALC PHOS: pain due to poor circulation
FERR PHOS: pain worse motion, muscular pain
NAT MUR: painful contractions of muscles

<u>How to look it up:</u>
CRAMPS: in limbs, pain, spasmodic
CLEANSER: removes poisons
CIRCULATION: parts feel cold
MUSCULAR: pain worse motion
MUSCULAR: painful contractions

The dosage is: 4 tablets of each four times a day dissolved under the tongue. Take at least 15 minutes away from food and drink.

## Case 2

The person is a 52-year-old female with the following symptoms:

• She has vertigo with blurred vision and flickering before the eyes.
• She feels very weak and afraid to drive because she thinks she will pass out.
• There are noises in her head with a feeling of confusion.

• She has had these symptoms for two weeks.
• She appears scared and desperate.

<u>The correct cell salts are:</u>

SILICA: for the vertigo
KALI PHOS: supports the nervous system
CALC FLUOR: flickering before the eyes

<u>How to look it up:</u>

VERTIGO: labyrinthitis
VISION: blurred
NERVES: primary cell salt
VISION: flickering before eyes

The dosage is 4 tablets of each of the four remedies four times a day dissolved under the tongue. Take at least 15 minutes away from food and drink.

# Case 3

A 39-year-old male presents very few symptoms:

• He wakes at 5 a.m. each morning and has to stretch excessively.
• He doesn't seem to have any control over it.
• This happens at least fifteen times each morning.
• He is tired all the time because of losing sleep each night.
• Sometimes parasites or worms can cause these types of symptoms.

<u>The correct cell salts are:</u>

FERR PHOS: is often indicated for restless sleep
NAT PHOS: balance any acidity causing brain irritation
MAG PHOS: for involuntary movements of muscles
KALI PHOS: for any nervous or muscular condition
CALC PHOS: is an anti-spasmodic

<u>How to look it up:</u>

SLEEP: restlessness, from worms
SLEEP: restlessness, in general
MUSCULAR: movements involuntary
YAWNING: and constant stretching

The dosage was given in liquid form as 10-15 drops three times a day. You can find liquid cell salts from some health-care practitioners. They are even easier to take.

# Case 4

A 28-year-old male complains of chronic rectal abscesses. The symptoms are:

• The rectal abscess fills with fluid and pus and then his doctor drains it.
• Over time the abscess fills up again.
• It has continued to do this for the last few years.
• The discharge is sticky and yellow.
• There is swelling of the surrounding tissue.

### The correct cell salts are:
CALC SULPH: blood cleanser and skin healer
CALC PHOS: for chronic abscesses
SILICA: brings discharge to the surface of the skin and also called the homeopathic surgeon

### How to look it up:
ABSCESS about anus
ABSCESS, chronic
ABSCESS, cleansing & healing
ABSCESS, helps when matter has formed
ABSCESS, ripen & suppurate, helps to
ABSCESS, clears up long standing
ABSCESS, promotes discharge
ABSCESS, sticky yellow discharge

The dosage is 4 tablets of each of the four remedies four times a day dissolved under the tongue. Take at least 15 minutes away from food and drink.

# BIBLIOGRAPHY

Boericke, William, M.D., and Willis A. Dewey, M.D., The Twelve Tissue Remedies of Schussler. 6th Ed., B. Jain Publishers Pvt. Ltd., New Delhi, India, 1985.

Carey, George W., M.D., The Chemistry of Human Life. The Chemistry of Life Co., Los Angeles, California, 1919.

Chapman, J.B., M.D., Dr. Schuessler's Biochemistry-A Natural Method of Healing. Thorsons Publishers Limited, Northamptonshire, England, 1982.

Chapman, J.B., M.D., and Dr. Edward L. Perry, M.D., The Biochemic Handbook, Formur, Incorporated, St. Louis, Missouri, 1976.

Ellingwood, Finley, M.D., American Materia Medica, Therapeutics and Pharmacognosy. Eclectic Medical Publication, Portland, Oregon, 1983.

Jackson, Mildred, N.D., and Terri Teague, N.D., The Handbook of Alternatives to Chemical Medicine. Self-Published, 1975.

Lepore, Donald, N.D., The Ultimate Healing System. Woodland Books, Provo, Utah, 1988.

Olshevshy, Moshe, C.A., Ph.D., S. Noy, M.D., M. Zwang, Ph.D. with R. Burger, The Manual of Natural Therapy: A Practical Guide to Alternative Medicine. Citadel Press, N.Y., N.Y., 1990.

Overton, Robert M., N.D., Schuessler's Tissue Remedies. Unpublished, 1985.

Powell, Eric F.W., PhD, N.D., Biochemic Prescriber. Health Science Press, Sussex, England. 1960.

Rector-Page, Linda, N.D., Ph.D., Healthy Healing: An Alternative Healing Reference. Spilman Printing, Sacramento, California, 1989.

Rolfe, Lionel, and Nigey Lennon, Natures's 12 Magic Healers-The Amazing Secrets of Cell Salts. Parker Publishing Company, Inc., West Nyack, New York, 1978.

Stein, Diane, The Natural Remedy Book for Women. The Crossing Press, Freedom, California, 1992.

Wendel, Dr. Paul, Homeopathic Materia Medica Condensed-The Twelve Remedies or Cell Salts of Dr. Schuessler. Dr. Paul Wendel Publishing, Brooklyn, N.Y.

# MEDICAL GLOSSARY

Aberrations....deviation from normal.

Acrid....burning, bitter, irritating.

Agglutination....clumping together, as of blood corpuscles when incompatible bloods are mixed; adhesion of surfaces or a wound.

Ague....used to indicate a chill or fever especially if due to malaria; rarely used today.

Albuminous....contains albumin; a group of simple proteins widely distributed in plant and animal ovalbumin. May refer to a discharge that resembles egg whites.

Alopecia....absence or loss of hair, especially of the head.

Ameliorated....improvement or moderation of a condition.

Amenorrhea....absence or suppression of menstruation.

Apparatus....a number of parts acting together in the performance of some special function; a group of structures or organs that work together to perform a common function.

Aneurysm....localized abnormal dilatation of a blood vessel usually an artery.

Apoplexy....cerebrovascular accident or stroke; usually thought of as a sudden loss of consciousness followed by paralysis caused by hemorrhage into the brain.

Areata....loss of hair in sharply defined patches usually involving the scalp or head.

Articulation....the place of union between two or more bones; a joint; may refer to speech.

Asphyxia....condition caused by insufficient intake of oxygen.

Asthenopia....weakness or tiring of eyes accompanied by pain, headache, and dimness of vision.

Atrophied....wasted; a decrease in size of an organ or tissue.

Balanitis....inflammation of the glans penis and mucous membrane beneath it; purulent discharge is usually present.

Biliousness....symptoms due to a disordered condition of the liver; excess of bile.

Blepharitis....inflammation of the edges of the eyelid involving hair follicles and glands that open onto the surface.

Bright's disease....a vague and obsolete term for disease of the kidneys; usually refers to inflammatory or degenerative kidney diseases characterized by protein and blood in the urine and sometimes edema, hypertension, and nitrogen retention.

Bursa....pad-like sac or cavity found in connecting tissue, usually in the
area of joints that contain a fluid.

Cachectic....a state of ill health, malnutrition, and wasting; may occur in
many chronic diseases. certain malignancies, and advanced pulmonary
tuberculosis.

Calcareous deposits....presence of calcium lime salts.

Calculi....usually a kidney stone or gallstone; any abnormal concretion
within the animal body; composed of mineral salts; can occur in the
kidneys, ureters, bladder, or urethra.

Canthi....the angle at either end of the slit between the eyelids.

Carditis....inflammation of the heart muscles.

Catarrh....inflammation of the mucous membranes especially of the head
and throat causing discharge.

Cerebral....the largest part of the brain consisting of two hemispheres separated by a deep longitudinal fissure.

Chancre....a hard, syphilitic primary ulcer; the first sign of syphilis appearing approximately two to three weeks after infection.

Chlorotic condition....a form of iron deficiency anemia.

Chorea....a nervous condition marked by involuntary muscular twitching
of the limbs or facial muscles.

Ciliary....usually pertaining to the eyelid, or any hair-like processes especially the eyelashes; to eye structures, such as the ciliary body.

Coitus....sexual intercourse; copulation.

Colic....spasm in any hollow or tubular soft organ accompanied by pain;
usually pertaining to the colon, but can occur in the bile duct associated with a gallstone, in the abdomen, kidneys, or in the uterus during the menstrual period.

Colitis....inflammation of the colon.

Condyles....a rounded protuberance at the end of a bone forming an articulation.

Conjunctiva....mucous membrane that lines the eyelids and is reflected
onto the eyeball.

Consolidation....the act of becoming solid; used in connection with the
solidification of the lungs due to pathological engorgement of the
lung tissues as occurs in acute pneumonia.

Corrosive....slow disintegration or wearing away of something by a destruc-
tive agent.

Coryza....an acute catarrhal inflammation of the nasal mucous membrane
accompanied by profuse nasal discharge.

Coxalgia....pain in the hip or hip joint disease.

Cretinism....congenital condition due to lack of thyroid secretion; characterized by arrested physical and mental development; the acquired form is called myxedema.

Derma....pertaining to the skin.

Dermal....pertaining to the skin.

Dermatoses....any disease of the skin where inflammation is not necessarily a feature.

Desquamation....shedding of the outer layer of skin.

Diathesis....constitutional predisposition to disease.

Diurnal....happening in the daytime or pertaining to it.

Dropsy....morbid accumulation of water in the tissues and cavities..

Duodenal....pertaining to the first part of the small intestines just beyond the stomach.

Dysentery....intestinal disorder especially of the colon; characterized by inflammation of the mucous membrane usually with abdominal pain, diarrhea, and passage of mucus or blood; may be caused by a bacterial or viral infection, protozoa, parasites, or by chemicals.

Dysmenorrhea....painful or difficult menses.

Dyspepsia....painful or imperfect digestion.

Dysphagia....inability or difficulty in swallowing.

Ecchymoses....a form of macula appearing in large irregularly formed hemorrhagic areas of the skin; the skin is blue-black changing to greenish-brown or yellow; blood seeping into the skin or mucous membranes.

Edema....a local or generalized condition where the body tissues contain an excessive amount of tissue fluid.

Emaciation....state of being extremely lean; malnutrition.

Embolism....obstruction of a blood vessel by foreign substances or blood clot.

Enchondroma....cartilaginous tumor.

Empyema....pus in a body cavity especially pleural cavity.

Endocarditis....inflammation of the membrane lining the heart.

Enervation....deficient in nervous energy; weakness.

Enteralgia....neuralgia or pain in the intestines relieved by bending double, warmth.

Enteric....pertaining to the small intestine.

Enteritis....inflammation of the intestines.

Enuresis....incontinence of urine.

Epididymitis....inflammation of a small oblong body resting upon and beside the posterior surface of the testes consisting of a convoluted tube 13-20 feet long.

Epiglottis....leaf-shaped structure located near the root of the tongue; covers the entrance of the larynx when individual swallows; prevents food or liquids from entering the airway.

Epithelioma....malignant tumor in the epidermis of the skin.

Epithelium....the layer of cells forming the outer surface of the skin and the surface layer of mucous and serous membranes.

Erethism, sexual....excessive excitement or irritation to stimuli.

Erysipelas....acute febrile disease with localized inflammation and redness of skin; subcutaneous tissue accompanied by a systemic disturbance; symptoms of fever, chills, nausea, vomiting, painful and warm skin, face and head lesions that are hot and red; usually caused by streptococcus pyogenes.

Excoriating....abrasion of the outer layer of the skin or of the coating of any organ of the body by trauma, chemicals, burns, or other causes.

Excrescence....the elimination of waste products from the body.

Exfoliation....the shedding of the human skin.

Exostosis....a bony growth that arises from the surface of a bone; often involving the ossification of muscular attachments.

Expectoration....spitting out saliva or coughing up material from the air passageways leading to the lungs.

Exudate....accumulation of a fluid in a cavity; matter that penetrates through vessel walls into adjoining tissue; the production of pus or serum.

Felon....infection or abscess of soft tissue of end joint of a finger; also called whitlow.

Fetid....rank or foul odor.

Fibrinous....containing fibrin—a whitish, filamentous protein formed by action of thrombin on fibrinogen; the basis for blood clotting.

Fistulous....abnormal tube-like passage from a normal cavity or tube to a free surface or to another cavity; may be due to congenital incomplete closure of parts, or may result from an abscess, injury, or inflammatory process.

Flatulence....excessive gas in the stomach and intestines.

Flocculent....a fluid or culture containing whitish shreds of mucus.

Fomentation....a hot, wet application for the relief of pain or inflammation; hot, moist dressing.

Fontanelles....an unossified space or soft spot lying between the cranial bones of the skull of a fetus or infant.

Glaucoma....disease of the eye characterized by an increase in intraocular pressure; can result in atrophy of the optic nerve and blindness.

Glottis....the sound producing apparatus of the larynx consisting of the two vocal folds and the intervening space.

Glycogenosis....abnormal accumulation of normal or abnormal forms of glycogen in tissue.

Glycogenolysis....conversion of glycogen into glucose in body tissues.

Granular....like granules or little grains.

Hemiopia....blindness in half of the visual field.

Hemoptysis....spitting up of blood from the oral cavity, larynx, trachea, bronchi, or lungs.

Hydrocele....accumulation of serous fluid in a sac-like cavity, especially in the testes or associated parts.

Hydrocephalus....increased accumulation of cerebrospinal fluid within the ventricles of the brain.

Hypochlorhydria....the diminished production of hydrochloric acid.

Hypochondriacal....abnormal anxiety about one's health; person fears or believes that they have a disease that persists despite medical reassurance that they do not.

Idiopathic....a primary disease without apparent cause.

Indolent....inactive, not developing, sluggish, indisposed to action; an indolent ulcer is slow to heal, but not painful.

Indurated....hardened; an area of hardened tissue.

Inguinal....pertaining to the region of the groin.

Insipid....without taste; lacking in spirit or animation.

Intercostal....between the ribs.

Intercurrent....intervening remedy.

Jaundice....condition characterized by the yellowness of the skin, whites of eyes, mucous membranes, and body fluids due to deposition of bile pigment; resulting from excess bilirubin in the blood.

Labia....the two folds of tissue lying on either side of the vaginal opening and forming the lateral borders of the vulva; pertains to the lips of the vaginal opening.

Lacrimal....pertaining to tears.

Lactation....the period of suckling in mammals; the function of secreting milk.

Lasciviousness....abnormal sexual desire; nymphomania.

Leukorrhea....usually white or yellow mucus discharge from the cervical canal or the vagina; usually indicates acute inflammation; discharge may be of any consistency.

Lithic....pertaining to uric acid that may be involved in stone formation.

Lumbago....a general non-specific term for dull, aching pain in the lumbar region of the back (low back pain).

Lymphadenopathy....disease of the lymph nodes.

Malassimilation....defective, incomplete, or faulty assimilation, especially of nutritive material; malabsorption syndrome.

Marasmus....emaciation and wasting in an infant due to malnutrition.

Mastitis....inflammation of the breast.

Mastoiditis....inflammation of the mastoid process; located on the skull behind the ear.

Meatus....a passage or opening usually referring to the ear canal, nasal passage, or opening to the bladder.

Meibomian glands....one of the sebaceous glands on the eyelids.

Mesenteric....a fold encircling the greater part of the small intestines and connecting the intestine to the posterior abdominal wall.

Necrosis....death of areas of tissue or bone surrounded by healthy parts.

Neuralgia....severe, sharp pain along the course of a nerve.

Neurasthenia....unexplained chronic fatigue and lassitude; usually accompanied by nervousness, irritability, anxiety, depression, headache, insomnia, and sexual disorders.

Noma....a gangrenous progressive condition, generally found in undernourished children, spreading rapidly from the mucous membrane of the cheek or gum to the skin surface.

Nystagmus....constant, involuntary, cyclical movement of the eyeball; movement may be in any direction.

Occipital....concerning the back part of the head.

Opaque....not transparent.

Optical....pertaining to vision or the eye.

Orchitis....inflammation of a testis due to trauma, cancer, mumps, or infection elsewhere in the body.

Osseous....bone-like; concerning the bones.

Ossification....formation of bone substance; conversion of other tissue into bone.

Osteophytes....a bony outgrowth usually branched in shape.

Ostitis....inflammation of a bone.

Otitis....an inflammation condition of the ear.

Ozena....disease of the nose characterized by atrophy of the inner membranes and considerable crusting, discharge, and a very offensive odor; present in various forms of rhinitis.

Palpitations....rapid, violent, or throbbing pulsation of the heart; abnormal fluttering of the heart; usually perceptible to the person.

Papular....concerning an eruption; usually a red elevated area on the skin, solid and with borders.

Parenchymatous....concerning the essential parts of an organ dealing with its function.

Paresis....partial or incomplete paralysis; organic mental disease with paralytic symptoms and running a chronic, slow, progressive course.

Paretic....affected with or concerning paresis.

Parotid gland....gland located near the ear and opens into the mouth; secretes fluid for the beginning process of digesting food; saliva.

Paroxysmal....occurring in or concerning a sudden, periodic attack or recurrence of symptoms of a disease; a worsening of the symptoms of a disease; a sudden spasm or convulsion of any kind.

Pedunculated....possessing a stalk or stem.

Pendulous....hanging; swinging freely like a pendulum.

Pericarditis....inflammation of the double membranous sac enclosing the heart.

Periosteum....the fibrous membrane that forms the covering of bones, except at the joint surface.

Peritonitis....inflammation of the peritoneum, the membranous coat lining the abdominal cavity.

Pharyngeal....concerning the pharynx; passageway for air from the nasal cavity to the larynx and for food from the mouth to the esophagus; also acts as a resonating cavity.

Phlebitis....inflammation of a vein with pain and tenderness along the course of the vein with discoloration of the skin along with edema.

Pleurisy....inflammation of the membrane that enfolds both of the lungs.

Posterior nares....the opening between the nasal cavity and the nasopharynx; the part of the air passageway situated above the soft palate; postnasal space; the nose.

Pott's disease....caries or osteitis of the vertebrae, usually of tuberculous origin; tubercular inflammation of bodies of the vertebrae; occurs primarily in children and in adults up to age 40.

Preputial....concerning the foreskin or fold of skin over the penis when circumcision has not occurred.

Purging....to evacuate the bowels by means of a substance that cleanses the bowels.

Purulent....full of pus.

Pustular....pertaining to a pustule; small elevation of skin filled with lymph or pus; may have defined border and be flat, rounded, or umbilicated.

Pylorus....opening between the stomach and the duodenum which is the first part of the small intestines.

Pyorrhea....a discharge of pus usually referring to a periodontal disease characterized by inflammatory or degenerative changes to the teeth and gums.

Pyrogenic....producing fever.

Quinsy....acute inflammation of the tonsil and surrounding area.

Remittent....alternately abating and returning at certain intervals as seen in some fevers.

Retinitis....inflammation of the retina of the eye.

Retracted....shortening; being drawn back.

Rhinitis....inflammation of the nasal mucosa with a congested condition of the nose and increased secretion of mucus; ozena; coryza; may be due to allergies.

Scapula....the shoulder blade.

Sciatica....severe pain in the leg along the course of the sciatic nerve; felt at the back of the thigh running down the inside of the leg.

Sclera....tough, white, fibrous tissue that covers the white of the eye.

Scrofulous....afflicted with a variety of tuberculosis that is most frequently encountered.

Scrotal....pertaining to the scrotum; the double pouch in the male that contains the testicles and part of the spermatic cord.

Secretion....the substance produced by glandular organs; material that flows out through a duct, such as saliva.

Senile....pertaining to the degenerative symptoms of old age.

Septic....pertaining to the presence of pathogenic bacteria in the blood; may cause infection; symptoms usually include chills, fever, and abscesses; blood poisoning.

Serous....having the nature of serum; producing a serum-like substance.

Spasmodic....concerning spasms.

Squamous....scale-like; squamous epithelium is a flat form of skin cells.

Strabismus....disorder of the eye where the optic axes cannot be directed to the same object; a squinting.

Subluxation....a partial or incomplete dislocation.

Submaxillary....pertaining to the upper jaw.

Suppuration....process of pus formation; the discharge produced by suppuration.

Supraorbital....located above the orbit of the eye.

Sycosis....chronic inflammation of hair follicles.

Synchondrosis....a joint become immovable; the cartilage eventually becomes ossified or permanently fixed.

Synovitis....inflammation of a part of the joint that contains lubricating fluid; painful joint, much more on motion, especially at night; swollen, skin sensitive to pressure.

Tabes dorsalis....a gradual, wasting, progressive, chronic disease of syphilis.

Tenacious....adhesive, tough.

Tepid....slightly warm; lukewarm.

Tetanic....pertaining to or producing tetanus; any agent producing tetanic spasms.

Tic douloureux....degeneration of or pressure on the trigeminal nerve resulting in neuralgia of that nerve. The pain comes on in severe lightning-like stabs and radiates from the angle of the jaw along one of the nerves.

Tinnitus....ringing, tinkling, buzzing or other sounds in the ear.

Torpidity....sluggishness, inactivity.

Tubercles....a small, rounded, elevation or eminence on a bone; small nodule on the skin or mucous membrane; characteristic lesion resulting from infection by tuberculosis.

Tympanic membrane....membrane serving as the eardrum.

Urethra....a canal for the discharge of urine extending from the bladder to the outside.

Urticaria....a vascular reaction of the skin characterized by the eruption of red wheals associated with severe itching; hives.

Varicocele....enlargement of the veins of the spermatic cord in the scrotum commonly occurring on the left side in adolescent males; dull ache along the cord; slight dragging sensation in the groin.

Vascular....pertaining to or composed of blood vessels.

Vertex of the head....top of the head.

Vesicle....a blister-like small elevation on the skin containing serous fluid.

Vesicular....pertaining to vesicles or small blisters.

Vexation....to agitate, to disturb, to annoy, to trouble seriously, or torment.

Viscid....adhering, glutinous, sticky.

Water brash....excessive saliva secreted in response to inflammation of the gastric mucous membrane.